Ketogenic Diet The Food Diary of a Fat Lad

Plus, a 30 Day Meal Diary and 100 Keto Recipes

Francis Devine

Table of Contents

87) Strawberry Basil Ice Cups

88) Blueberry Ice cream

89) Apple-Apricot Cloud

90) Creamy Peanut Butter Dessert

91) Lime Mousse

92) Rich Chocolate Muffin

93) Chocolate Cherry Cheesecake

94) Cinnamon Churritos:

95) Vanilla Crème Pudding Parfaits

96) Pumpkin Spice Crème Brule

97) Strawberry Cheesecake Fat Bombs

98) Lemon Cheesecake Pudding

99) Mocha Ice cream

100) Mint and Chocolate Chip Ice Bombs

Chapter One: Dave's Fat Lad Manifesto

This is a story about Dave, our roommate. He put on twenty kilos in the last three years. Now, his doctor is saying that he might get diabetes if he doesn't make a change.

We put this book together because Dave needed help, and he wouldn't get it done on his own because of a lack of motivation and a general sense of, "I've tried it all and nothing works." So, we asked him to write a diary for us so we could look through it every few days to help him with his eating habits and his general health.

We also told him we would do it with him in the beginning, just to help him get started.

We wanted Dave to set his own goals for us in writing, so he couldn't back out. So, we asked him to spend some time thinking about goals so he could write them out on paper. We also thought he should write out his inner thoughts and motivations in order to help keep him on track.

He rambles sometimes, but that's mostly because he doesn't want to be writing a diary. He thinks it's stupid, and wants us to drop the subject. But, we figure a journal is going to help him in the long run because he can visibly see his journey in a format that is familiar to him. He writes professionally, so we figured this type of progress charting would help him.

He keeps trying to dodge us, though, so we got him to promise us he would stick to the plan for four months.

Day 1

Ok. So, the guys are making me write this dumbass journal. I'm convinced it's because they want something to make fun of in a couple months when everything fails.

Maybe not. Francis seems to be genuine when he offers his help.

Anyway. They're buying my beers tonight. That's how they convinced me to keep this diary. They want me to write every day, but we'll just have to see on that one.

So... yeah. Why I'm doing this. Well, I'm done being uncomfortable with my weight, and I just put on too much over the last few years. I think it started in my early twenties, but the bulk of my weight gain happened over the last three or four years.

I can't really pinpoint when, but I'm guessing it's when I started eating "better," when I could afford a decent meal instead of simply living off instant noodles. I also stopped eating junk food (except during hangovers) and basically ate more because I could afford more.

The big jump was when I was with my last girlfriend, though. We would spend so much time being lazy at home, or sitting on the couch and watching shows. We'd even cook things together... you know, get creative with recipes and stuff. That's when I started enjoying making food, and between always cooking it and always being lazy, I just put on weight. I even stopped going out at night and dancing, which was my only workout. I guess it was the domestication that lead to a sedentary lifestyle. It wasn't even her fault, so I can't blame her for it. I would insist we stayed home. She tried to get me out of it, after the first ten kilos happened, but it was a bit late then. I was firmly set in my habits.

So, with her I gained fifteen kilos. Not really because of her, but I like to blame her for it sometimes. Helps me cope, I guess.

Also, it's annoying to take the stairs. It's frustrating to walk around for too long, and sometimes it's even difficult to just sit in some places. But, the most annoying thing is always having to dish out money for new clothes when I outgrow what I have. I just can't do that anymore.

The doctor says my blood sugar levels are high and I need to watch out for my health in the future 'cause my uncle's got diabetes, so that's another looming threat to my health.

Apparently, this ketogenic stuff is a good way to deal with sugar levels. The doc recommended it and the guys looked into it. Seems like it should work. So, I'm into it, for now.

That means it's time to chill. Aside from that, it'd be good to feel happy about the way I look again. It's been years since I looked in the mirror and didn't try to suck my stomach in. Also, man boobs -they don't suit me

So, goals. They told me to write down goals and motivations.
- → *I will drop between three and five kilos each month.*
- → *I will listen to what Francis and Jared say –regarding food– when I falter for four months.*
- → *I will make sure to keep my sugar intake to a minimum.*
- → *I will not bitch about the way I look to girls anymore (yea, right).*
- → *I will go dancing every week.*
- → *I will start walking around the city again.*
- → *I will not allow Francis and Jared to force me to work out, ever.*

- → *I will not allow Francis and Jared to deny me basic alcohol intake on a weekly basis.*
- → *I will not allow Francis and Jared to bitch about the way I look until after the diet is over.*
- → *I will not allow Francis and Jared to starve me if they're not also starving with me.*

There we go. That should be it. I'll sign this like the lads asked, but seriously, if this gets out of hand, I'm having a few pints and relaxing!

And that was it. We had it in writing. We all signed it and got to work. We'd heard great success stories, so we were ready to give it a go. For our buddy, you know?

While waiting for Dave to write up his diary entry and negotiate his manifesto, it dawned on Jared and myself. We would have to commit to doing this for two months.

Dave had good reason to lose weight and we were being supportive friends, but we were not the dieting type. Jared is a fitness buff, so he eats whatever he wants. I enjoy taking life as it comes and don't really bother with diets or anything like that.

The day before we had to start, Jared pulled me aside and started discussing ways that we could keep tabs on each other during this diet. I look back now and realize that none of it turned out to be necessary. It was easy to keep to the diet because it was… fun. Sometimes, we drank more than we should've, but we weren't worried about the empty calories.

You know, youthful ignorance and all.

Chapter Two: What is a Ketogenic Diet?

The idea of ketosis is simple and the ketogenic diet is built around concepts that by and large make sense to the average person. Eat lean food, keep the sugar and carbohydrate intake to a minimum, and don't snack every time you want to.

Reaching ketosis is useful because it is the state of chemical balance that makes the body use up any residual fat in your system. It is fooled into thinking it's not getting enough food due to the low carb intake. Basically, your body thinks it's starving, and protects itself.

The thing is, you're not actually starving yourself. Yes, you are cutting carbohydrates down to less than forty grams a day, sometimes even below twenty, but you're still eating quite a bit. You have no limit on the amount of fat you can consume.

The only other trick is to moderate your protein intake: keep it to around one gram of protein per kilogram of your desired weight. Add that up and you're still eating more than enough to feel satiated.

The other thing about "going keto" is that it makes you less hungry. You're eating more calories than normal, not less. But, outside the lack of sugar and the volume reduction in food intake, there is something else that is usually overlooked: most ketogenic diets recommend intermittent daily fasts usually on 16:8 or 20:4 cycles. What does that mean? One of the first things that we did when we heard about intermittent fasting was to look it up, and it turns out that intermittent fasting can be quite easy to follow.

A 16:8 fast basically means that you allow yourself a window of 8 hours of eating during a 24-hour cycle (skip breakfast and have an early dinner, with food in between). The 20:4 cycle is a bit more difficult, but not unheard of, if you've got a really busy work day.

You eat nothing outside of the eating window. During the food window, you stick to your ketogenic habits.

It's not just great for weight loss. A ketogenic diet is also great for treating diabetics and reducing the risk of diabetes among those prone to it. This is because of the super low sugar intake.

It's also excellent for people at risk for heart disease. A ketogenic diet helps with blood pressure regulation, balancing blood sugars, and reducing body fat percentage. It helps with acne, cancer, Alzheimer's, epilepsy, Parkinson's, polycystic ovary syndrome, and even brain injuries.

The benefits that you can get from the diet and the conclusiveness of the research regarding specific health benefits is still largely open to debate. We'll get into that in a later chapter.

Before we began our keto experiment, we decided to break down the food groups to see how much we'd actually be giving up.

Foods to avoid

Avoiding foods which are "high in carbs" seems straightforward enough, but there's got to be a catch somewhere, right? It can't just be avoiding french fries, sodas, bread, and sweets. And there was indeed a little more to it:

Say no to fruits. Even though fruits are a natural source of sugar, they still contain a lot of sugar. A tiny portion of berries might be okay, but that's it. Juice is an especially bad idea, even if it's freshly squeezed with no additives. And, you have to make sure to stay away from sugar additives. If the label says, "sugar free,", think twice about eating it. This label is often assigned to processed foods with unnatural artificial sweeteners that can prevent your body from going into ketosis.

Say no to those so called "healthy snacks" such as beans, carrots, parsnips, lentils, and chickpeas. While these foods are preferable to a big bucket of soda, all of these have a ton of carbs.

Say no to sauces. Unless you make them yourself, stay away. You need to hold the ketchup, drop the mayo, and avoid vegetable oils. And, you should definitely drop most processed, non-naturally sourced food items.

Say no to alcohol. Well, not all alcohol, but fruity cocktails and beers are out of the question, which was a massive bummer to myself and the guys. Wine is alright since the carbohydrate count is much lower in them, and so are spirits, in case you're wondering. Just make sure to avoid the overly sweet wines.

What is good keto food, then?

Meat. Any meat. Fish as well, especially the fatty types like salmon, tuna, mackerel, and trout. Eggs, butter, cream, cheese, nuts, seeds, healthy oils, non-starchy vegetables, herbs, spices, and superfoods like avocados are good for the diet, too.

Try sticking to simple meals. Just eggs, just beef, just bacon, just chicken, just asparagus, just cucumber, just mushrooms. You get the idea. Often times, the less you add to it, the better it's going to be. Of course, when I say "just", I mean you can still add spices, herbs, salt, and pepper.

Steam them, fry them (only in extra virgin olive oil or coconut oil), or grill them, but don't slather them in those additive-filled, carbohydrate-heavy sauces.

The simplicity recommended in keto diets makes it easier to prepare a lot of the foods, and for variety you can simply mix and match. For some people, it's not really a major lifestyle change, as their normal eating habits are focused on these basic food items and they already cook simply.

The biggest challenge tends to be in the things to avoid. Or, at least, it would seem so at first. For Dave, it was easy. He only had pasta about once or twice a month. It was beer and bread that he needed to drop. The rest of his food intake was pretty much "keto" already. His diet was too heavy on beer and bread.

Focus on minimizing ingredients

Keep meals to less than 4 items each, and cook them in as few pots and pans as possible. Also, eat enough to feel satisfied, but keep it all to one reasonably sized plate.

For example, you might have a shrimp salad with olive oil and avocado. Consider an egg omelet for breakfast, maybe with mushrooms and cheese, or bacon and onions. Chicken wrapped in serrano ham, stuffed with garlic cream cheese, with a side of spinach for dinner. Sounds pretty tasty, right?

Remember to keep cycling through food items. It's important to get a mix of nutrients from different things. It also keeps you from getting bored on the diet.

Dining out or ordering in?

Most restaurants have lots of keto friendly meals. It's also easy to modify a meal to be low carb. But, when you can't, there are some tricks you can have up your sleeve. Have a burger with the bun but hold the fries, or ditch the bun and splurge on the fries. Or, if you're really trying to stick to it strictly, ditch the bun and get some veggies on the side.

When in doubt, a steak meal works perfectly. A lot of salads are fine, too. And egg-based meals are fantastic.

What about side effects and supplements?

Being tired while at work was not an option for us. We needed to remain alert and energized. We were also worried that the lack of fruits in our diet could be problematic or that we might have other unexpected side effects.

We were right. Sort of.

When you first start a ketogenic diet, your body will try to adapt. You will need to give it a few days while it deals with the change. Your body may respond by becoming rather lethargic during this time.

You'll be low on energy, hungry often, nauseous sometimes, and maybe even struggle with sleep. There could also be some degree of digestive problems or fatigue. Your body needs to go through this weakened state for it to activate ketosis and become familiar with the new substance your body will burn in order to get its energy. Fat! Some recommended going for a low-carb diet before going full keto but we decided to just dive right in.

The other thing we wondered about were supplements. They're not required, but hey, if you'd like to try some, nobody's stopping you. In fact, your body's minerals will reshuffle themselves during and after the keto adaptation period, so it might be wise.

Common supplements include MCT oil, minerals, and even ketone supplements and whey protein. Creatine and caffeine were the ones that really stood out for us though.

Caffeine from coffee is generally part of a ketogenic diet anyway, as long as you don't add sugar and you keep your milk or cream balanced. We drank a lot of coffee as it was intended to counter the initial fatigue and lower energy levels. Bulletproof coffee is a popular keto concoction consisting of coconut oil or MCT oil and unsalted butter, blended into black coffee. It tastes amazing and is an excellent way to consume healthy fat.

Creatine is a great supplement that also has a lot of health benefits. It's especially useful for people who are still running a full work-out regimen while on a ketogenic diet. It keeps your body from dropping muscle mass, keeps your strength up and generally helps you stay active.

Remember that thing about fasting?

There was another lifestyle adjustment that really changed things up during our keto experiment. We're still debating now if it was really the one thing that made all the difference or not.

We lived by a 16:8 system for our entire two-month period. Dave sustained it for the entire six months. Sometimes, we'd even go for the 20:4 window. Dave told us he experimented with a 48:24 protocol, which basically means eating only every other day.

To Recap:

- Ketosis is a state where your body doesn't get enough carbs and so it burns the fat in your body as its primary fuel source.
- A ketogenic diet has numerous health benefits. Particularly those related to the heart, the liver and mental function, but also certain cancers and skin problems.
- Meal plans are easy to follow and tend to fit comfortably with most people's eating habits and the sort of dishes served at the majority of restaurants.
- Drinking alcohol will require some changes (no more beer) but it's still quite simple to substitute lower carb wine or spirits.
- There is a recommended system of fasting that involves restricting food intake to certain hours of the day, which is both good for your health and easy to manage (also, you don't do it all the time).
- Side effects are usually only at the start, and are easily mitigated with some basic supplements, which are optional.
- You don't really need supplements during your diet because you're mostly eating the same foods as always.
- A lot of these points need further elaboration, which we'll get to in subsequent chapters.

First, let's discuss the meal plans that we came up with.

Chapter Three: A Meal Plan to Start

It is recommended by specialists that you start with a strict two-to-four- week ketogenic eating schedule, to get your body used to the program, before you allow yourself a more flexible eating schedule. This acts as a vehicle to aid in the development of a new habit. After a few weeks, your body will become adapted to the change and you can better regulate eating for yourself. The general rule of thumbs goes as such: we needed to take in one gram of protein for every kilo of our targeted body weight. We needed to keep our carb intake under 40 grams a day, and we needed to make sure that our fat intake to carb intake ratio was always 4:1.

So, we did exactly that. We stuck to the regimen outlined for us before we started to take our own dietary liberties. Some people do a three-day kick-starter, others do two weeks. It's up to you, but we wanted the full effect as quickly as possible.

We decided that each day would involve three meals, and that we'd leave the snacking for when it was necessary. We decided to give ourselves three days of 16:8 fasts every 9-10 days. For Dave, we turned one of the three day fasts into a 20:4 day (so there would only be two meals that day).

It was easy. We sat in the kitchen one day with lots of paper and a bottle of wine and planned out our food for the next 30 days.

We love eggs. So, we designed four different omelets and mixed them up during the week. We also had coffee breakfasts or just fried or scrambled eggs with bacon on the side. Day six would be the start of our 3-day fast but that wouldn't be consistent throughout the month. And we cycled between chicken, beef, seafood, turkey, pork, and shellfish every six days, with one no-meat day a week.

We're usually big drinkers, so we scheduled our drinking habits, too. At first, we had a strict schedule for our limited booze We weren't very good at keeping to the schedule. But, we maintained the amount of drinks we'd allowed ourselves, and never went over. You'd probably have better results if you did not follow our drinking advice. Dave limited his alcohol intake a lot after the first month, and his results were much better than ours in the beginning.

We quickly discovered that our alcohol tolerance was much lower on the ketogenic diet, so be wary of that when you get into it. Drink more slowly so you can keep track of how you feel.

This chapter is about how we set up the meal plan but it's also about how the keto experiment all went down. Dave will have his own take on it in his diary entry later, but we also went through it. Although we weren't looking to lose as much weight as he was - we felt the effects.

Round 1: The First 10 Days

We were a bit worried that, since it's our first week, we'd be dealing with general keto adjustment issues, especially hunger. So, we planned out larger meals that we could reheat in order to conserve energy and get used to this new change.

Before you jump in, there's another little detail: we didn't always have the lunch and dinner options in the right order. Sometimes, we'd have dinner instead of lunch because it was the three of us and we felt like swapping. We didn't feel like it would be a problem, and it wasn't.

Day 1
- Breakfast: bacon and mushroom omelet with coriander sprinkles.
- Lunch: chicken casserole with olives and feta cheese in pesto sauce.
- Dinner: grilled beef fillet in peppercorn sauce with sautéed spinach on the side.

Day 2
- Breakfast: scrambled eggs with chopped avocado in garlic, lemon, and olive oil.
- Lunch: salmon with fried asparagus cooked in butter. Glass of white wine.
- Dinner: leftover chicken casserole with olives and feta cheese in pesto sauce.

Day 3
- Breakfast: Bulletproof coffee (Coffee with butter and MCT oil).
- Lunch: pork stir fry in coconut oil.
- Dinner: wine night, with a cheese and cold cuts platter. Probably a bottle each.

Day 4
- Breakfast: BLT sandwich with black coffee (no sugar).
- Lunch: Thai coconut curry with white fish.
- Dinner: cheese pimiento meatballs with steamed broccoli on the side.

Day 5
- Breakfast: egg, cheese, and onion omelet with tomatoes.
- Lunch: leftover cheese pimiento meatballs with steamed broccoli on the side.
- Dinner: roast turkey slices with a thick cream sauce.

At this point, the keto adaptation period had passed because it would normally kick in between the third and fifth day, which is why we decided to not fast until then. So, the big attack on our energy levels would come from the first fasting period. We planned these meals in a way so that time between snacks made sense, so we'd actually eat it (and actually feel full enough for/during the fast). Then, on our last day of fasting, we decided that getting a bit drunk and starting our next day with a hefty breakfast would be a good idea.

Day 6 (16:8)
- Breakfast: Greek yogurt with cocoa and peanut butter.
- Lunch: bacon-wrapped meatloaf.
- Dinner: cabbage, ground beef, ginger, garlic, and other spices, all in a stir fry.

Day 7 (20:4)
- Brunch: bacon, mushroom, tomato, onion, and cheese-egg omelet with herbs and spices.
- Dinner: Bulletproof coffee to wrap up the day and help avoid hunger pangs. Maybe leftover meatloaf if hungry.

Day 8 (16:8)
- Breakfast: salmon poached eggs on a bed of sautéed spinach.
- Lunch: avocado, bacon, and shrimp salad with a light vinaigrette dressing. Glass of white wine.
- Dinner: cheese & cold-cuts snack. Wine night.

Day 9
- Breakfast: scrambled eggs with olives, diced halloumi and pancetta. Garnished with parsley.
- Lunch: leftover roast turkey slices, and leftover avocado, bacon, and shrimp salad with the rest of the light vinaigrette dressing.
- Dinner: oven baked garlic, lemon, and parsley chicken.

Day 10
- Breakfast: Bulletproof coffee.
- Lunch: leftover garlic chicken with a side of cauliflower mash.
- Dinner: grilled beef fillet with cauliflower mash. Red wine night.

After our first fast, we figured it would be clever to keep our intake a bit on the low end. So, day nine was a binge day, but day ten slowed it down again before going into round two. You'll notice we tried to experiment with various dishes but, at some point, just cycled back towards familiar meals.

In most cases, we realized you don't need to have more than a 10-day meal plan as you could just cycle meals around from the ten-day plan. But just to be super sure, the three of us knew what was going on and we got into ketosis, we kept a full month's calendar. Besides, Dave isn't big on eating the same thing too often.

Round Two: 10 More Days

We looked up a few really cool recipes for low-carb rice replacements, so we thought we'd try them out over the course of these ten days. A big one is cauliflower and another is cabbage.

Day 1
- Breakfast: two fried eggs with bacon on the side.
- Lunch: bun-less cheeseburger with bacon and tomatoes.
- Dinner: cauliflower soup with pancetta.

Day 2
- Breakfast: scrambled eggs with chopped avocado in garlic, lemon, and olive oil.
- Lunch: leftover cauliflower soup.
- Dinner: pork chops with cucumber Greek yogurt salad.

Day 3
- Breakfast: Bulletproof coffee.
- Lunch: beef stroganoff with cauliflower rice.
- Dinner: cheese pimiento meatballs with steamed broccoli on the side. Wine night.

Dave didn't want to wait too long before he did a second fast period, because it just made sense to keep the rhythm. We decided to jolt our bodies into two, consecutive 20:4 days. Eggs keep us full - so we went with that. Also, we realized that we can just drink coffee during the fasting hours, so we made proper food in between.

Dave actually ended up rescheduling Day 3 so that it was a 20:4 but we stuck to the original program.

Day 4 (20:4)
- Brunch: savory low-carb pancakes with garlic cream cheese on top.
- Dinner: bacon, mushroom, tomato, onion, and cheese-egg omelet, with herbs and spices.

Day 5 (20:4)
- Brunch: grilled steak with a Mexican omelet.
- Dinner: fried chicken with aioli sauce to dip.

Right out of the fast period, we didn't want to overdo it on the food, so we kept it simple. Some leftovers from a few days prior made a convenient meal. Then, since we had planned on avoiding the fast for a week, we could get back into our drinking habits.

We noticed that we hadn't really assigned a lot of seafood to the meal plan this week, so we crammed it all in because seafood is a great addition a ketogenic diet.

At this point, two weeks in, we were actually starting to notice the difference in our bodies. The weight loss, the general energy, and certainly our reduced appetite were all pleasant consequences of our efforts. We were more alert at work, and gym time just flowed more smoothly. All the advertised health benefits were starting to kick in. Except the skin benefits, but then again, we weren't quite sure what the best way to measure that was.

We all experienced the weight change though. Dave dropped 3 kilos in just those two weeks, and we all felt a little less flabby. There were decent results overall.

Day 6
- Breakfast: breakfast tapas (basically, olives, cold cuts, and cheese).
- Lunch: leftover cheese pimiento meatballs with steamed broccoli on the side.
- Dinner: wine night with a cheese and cold cuts platter.

Day 7
- Breakfast: scrambled eggs with olives, diced halloumi and pancetta. Garnished with parsley.
- Lunch: leftover fried chicken.
- Dinner: pork and shrimp stir fry with cabbage rice.

Day 8
- Breakfast: Greek yogurt with cocoa and peanut butter.
- Lunch: salmon cooked in butter with cabbage rice. Glass of white wine.
- Dinner: roast turkey slices with a thick cream sauce.

Day 9
- Breakfast: coconut porridge.
- Lunch: leftover roast turkey slices with a simple avocado salad as a side.
- Dinner: cabbage, ground beef, ginger, garlic, and other spices all in a stir fry.

Day 10
- Breakfast: Bulletproof coffee.
- Lunch: Thai coconut curry with white fish. White wine.
- Dinner: chicken casserole with olives and feta cheese in pesto sauce.

And, that was a wrap. The benefits of our ketogenic diet experiment looked very promising. We all agreed that it felt fantastic. It was easy to maintain. We didn't always stick to the meal plan at this stage (we couldn't be bothered to make the curry for the white fish on day ten), so we just grilled it and had some of the leftover stir fry from dinner the night before. There was no leftover fried chicken so we just grilled some breaded chicken strips. Overall, we were on our game.

Round Three: Twenty Days Down, Ten to Go.

For the last stretch, we looked up many different recipes and tried to simplify them, so we wouldn't always need the recipe in front of us in order to cook them. We got a bit creative and more intense in this round with the fasting as well, and pushed our limits to see how far we could go. You'll also notice a favorite of ours during the 20:4 fast, the "Everything- In Omelet." It kept us full for the rest of the day. Also, we fasted for longer this time.

Overall, it was a productive ten days. We dropped our drinking down to just once during the ten days, but Dave was still convinced that it wasn't necessary even when we did it. We tended to agree. We were feeling great.

Day 1
- Breakfast: egg sausage cakes made in a pan with dark greens, onions, parsley, and other fresh herbs added to eggs and a couple cups of sausage filling.
- Lunch: ground beef mixed with spices and spinach leaves cooked in coconut oil with sliced bell peppers on the side.
- Dinner: meatballs done Moroccan style with either cauliflower or cabbage rice on the side.

Day 2
- Breakfast: coconut porridge.
- Lunch: leftover egg sausage cakes.
- Dinner: chicken, bacon, lettuce, tomato, and hard-boiled egg salad with a light dressing.

This was the five- day fast we were all slightly worried about. It risked being a bit too much for us, but we could always just cheat with a small snack, or just drink coffee to suppress our appetites. We had been told that by the time we'd been on the keto diet for this long that we wouldn't really feel as hungry anymore, so we decided to give it a try.

It was true. We didn't get hungry. In fact, it was almost easy. Our other concern was being tired during all the cycles, but that also wasn't a problem. Don't get me wrong, though, it wasn't easy making it through that last day.

Day 3 (20:4)
- Brunch: bacon, mushroom, tomato, onion and cheese egg omelet with herbs and spices.
- Dinner: leftover Moroccan meatballs with leftover chicken BLT salad.

Day 4 (20:4)
- Brunch: bacon and eggs - lots of them.
- Dinner: curried shrimp with cabbage rice.

Day 5 (16:8)
- Breakfast: your choice of eggs scrambled with your choice of veggies and meats cooked in coconut oil.
- Lunch: grilled fish with a simple side of greens.
- Dinner: fried chunks of chicken breast cooked with shredded cheddar and chopped garlic.

Day 6 (16:8)
- Breakfast: bulletproof coffee.
- Lunch: bun-less cheeseburger.
- Dinner: cheese pimiento meatballs with steamed broccoli on the side.

Day 7 (20:4)
- Brunch: garlic cream cheese stuffed chicken breasts wrapped in Serrano ham with a side of cabbage mash.
- Dinner: cold cuts and cheese platter with red wine.

Day 8
- Breakfast: Greek yogurt with cocoa and peanut butter.
- Lunch: mustard lime marinated butterfly chicken.
- Dinner: breaded fish sticks with coleslaw on the side.

Day 9
- Breakfast: bacon and mushroom omelet with coriander sprinkles.
- Lunch: chicken casserole with olives and feta cheese in pesto sauce.
- Dinner: grilled beef fillet in peppercorn sauce with sautéed spinach on the side.

Day 10
- Breakfast: scrambled eggs with chopped avocado in garlic, lemon and olive oil.
- Lunch: salmon with fried asparagus cooked in butter. Glass of white wine.
- Dinner: leftover chicken casserole with olives and feta cheese in pesto sauce.

And, there you go. That's all 30 days of our fantastic keto eating journey. You can even make up your own. We made up a few of these as we went along. It's all about the right ingredients put together in a way that ensures that your carb intake is as low as possible - all the time. Making sure your fat and protein intake is high enough is also key to promoting ketosis.

Remember:
- Keep your carb intake under 40 grams, but get it lower if you can.
- Take in at least one gram of protein for every kilo of your desired weight (so, if you want to be 81 kilos, you need to eat 81 grams of protein).
- Whatever the numbers are, make sure the ratio is at least 4:1 for your fat intake to carb intake ratio.

Chapter Four: Dear Diary

Well, here is Dave's diary. He really did try, although I'm not sure he utilized it to the furthest extent that he could have. But, we did get him to use it, and we think it did help him to jot down his feelings during the entire first 30 days. He might not admit it, but we saw him think through his lifestyle choices more as the days progressed.

But, don't tell him that. He's convinced it didn't work.

Day 1

I don't know why they want me writing every day. There's nothing to say. Food was awesome. It's normal food. I imagine it'll get harder once we hit the fasting periods and when I get random cravings for sandwiches or fries or... carby things.

Day 2

The salmon was awesome! I'd never had fried asparagus before. Usually only steamed. It was nice. Other than that? Still a normal day.

Day 3

Bulletproof coffee is pretty interesting... I'd never had it before. It's intense. Definitely kept me full and energized though. And if only wine nights happened all the time. Then I'd be happy.

Day 4

Again, this is fun. Nothing new to add. I think I'm starting to get what they mean about pissing too often when you're on keto though. It's been way too often. I also feel a bit sleepy. But my brain is more active which is cool, I guess. Let's see.

Day 5

Yup. Definitely in ketosis now. The guys are saying they feel different, the normal everyday bloating they had is totally gone. I think it's just a bit gone. I want beer but I know I should behave.

Day 6

I was worried about today. This low carb yogurt nonsense isn't usually for me but it was a good light meal that I packed with me to work. The meatloaf was also easy to carry to work. Made sure to have them only 3 hours apart and then had dinner three hours later too. 16:8 is not so bad.

On a different note, I'm not sure I've lost weight (we agreed I'd only weigh myself once a month), but I do feel better. Like I might actually be slimming a bit. I think it's in my head though. Let's see…

Day 7

Okay, 20:4 is not fun. That omelet was incredible though. Had it around lunch time. Kept myself sane throughout with tea. And damn that Bulletproof coffee stuff works! I really want beer. Wine tomorrow! I cheated and had a glass today though.

Day 8

Yes, for wine!! It was a great tap on the back, me thinks. Cheers to you, Francis and Jared.

Day 9

I like tea a lot. I can definitely see body changes. I'm not hallucinating. I couldn't stop talking about it tonight. Might have been the whiskey. Had four of those.

Day 10

Still tea. I didn't know cauliflower mash could taste so good. Also, ouch, hangover. Why can't I just beer my way through this?

Day 11

They made me eat a burger without a bun. I only agreed to do it because they agreed to post a photo of all three of us eating one on Facebook. Cheers to whiskey, again. I'm liking this.

Day 12

Just so you know, I'm not writing these every day. I'm filling them in retrospectively. Still, accurate though. I think my belly is shrinking on a daily basis now. Like, I'm certain of it. The guys think I'm delusional. I'll show them delusional.

Day 13

They want to start the fast tomorrow but I figured I'd start a day early cause this weight loss stuff is making sense. So, I skipped breakfast and lunch, just had dinner and made sure I didn't drink too much wine (three glasses and I stopped —no, wait, four). Made it into a 20:4 day.

Day 14

Those pancakes are yummy. I am so glad that I can drink as much tea as I want during these fasts.

Day 15

Fried chicken. Yum. Need more of that in my life. Also had whiskey tonight. Lots of it. Apparently, that's allowed, because it's got zero carbs.

Day 16

This was a 16:8 day by mistake. Didn't go to the office today and slept in, so breakfast and lunch kind of just meshed together. Then wine night was fun.

Day 17

Okay I must have lost at least five kilos already! I've got trousers that didn't used to fit me that do now, and my everyday jeans are getting a bit loose. Even though I just got them out of the dryer. I pulled out an old favorite pair I hadn't worn in like two years. When I was seven kilos lighter, they were tight. Now they fit me like a glove. Maybe this is a good thing!

Day 18

Good food. Still excited about my weight loss. Really want to weigh myself, but promised not to. Thought about sneaking a pint but had a whiskey instead. It actually works out drinking whiskey because it makes you look all posh and shit.

Day 19

I actually couldn't finish my plate today. The stir-fry. I felt defeated! That's a first!

Day 20

Okay, now it's a second. The casserole was delicious but even one portion was too much. I think I read about this somewhere... you kind of stop being as hungry because you get used to less food. Also, that Bulletproof coffee. I like it. I should have it more often.

Day 21

I had fun making those egg sausage cakes. Next month, I'll make them more often. Francis made lunch. Jared wasn't allowed into the kitchen. He's burnt food before. Went out to celebrate with the lads. We all drank whiskey instead of pints. I could get used to this.

Day 22

So, made this into a 16:8 day, cause I'm trying to push myself more than the guys need to for their own plan. It was easy, I just skipped the porridge. Not really a fan anyway.

Day 23

20:4 day. I love that omelet. So, yum. The meatballs also tasted better two days later.

Day 24

Tea day. Only way I managed to survive the 20:4 today. I then had one whiskey at night but I worry about drinking too much on fast days. It's like drinking on an empty stomach. Note to self: don't do that again!

Day 25

The win was the fried chicken. I think there should be fried chicken on every 16:8 day. Also, it was an awesome recipe! It's just so easy, even Jared could make it. We wouldn't have found out if he hadn't snuck into the kitchen and made it just to prove a point.

Day 26

I can't believe I'm eating bun less burgers, but considering the way I feel and look at the moment, it's soooooo worth it! Also, today was a 16:8 day but the Bulletproof coffee in the morning helped.

Day 27

That day's recipe was a creation of mine from last year. Except the mash. I used to use actual garlic mashed potatoes. Still worked with the cabbage though. And then we drank to seal off the 20:4!

Day 28

Okay, so I had to eat a lot more for lunch because of my hangover so I had lunch and dinner at the same time. Made it a 20:4 day though not on purpose. Peppermint tea saved me the rest of the day. That makes for a whole week of intermittent fasting!! And just at the end of the month, too, so my numbers are bound to look awesome. Yes baby, yes!

Day 29

Oh, it's so good to eat so much again! It was my idea to go back to heavier food the way we started the month. Needed it.

Day 30

And I got to weigh myself today. You won't believe the numbers.

I started off at 84kg. I'm now at 78kg!! That's a six kilo drop! It feels more like ten, to be honest. But, I'll trust the numbers. This is definitely working. And it was easy. Fun, even!

During the entire month, it felt like a game... not a diet. I was still eating most things and still drinking normally. I was impressed with the way that the diet made me less hungry and gave me a lower appetite, I was also just eating smaller portions.

I did have some beer cravings that I wasn't really satisfying, but that wasn't so hard. Swap it in with wine and I'm a happy chap. The fact that the diet made it easier for me to drink less because I'd get tipsy faster certainly had a massive impact on my caloric intake, too. The guys warned me about this, and so had the Google.

Next month I think I'll drink less. Tonight though, I'm celebrating! I think a few glasses of whiskey will do…

In a departure from my usual routine, I stopped taking public transport and started using my bike more often. Almost always, actually. When I didn't cycle around town, I walked. I used my step counting app on my phone to make sure I did over thirty thousand steps a day, trying to increase that to over fifty thousand on the weekends because that meant I was burning more calories.

And, the other super important thing - I think my blood sugar is balancing out, too. I don't want to check it because I don't want to feel like I'm a sick person. I'll know when I see my doctor next week. Hopefully, I won't have to see him about my weight again anytime soon.

Chapter Five: Progress for the Rest of Us

Dave's keto weight loss story was a success. And I'm happy to say that the progress that Jared and I made over the course of the other three months was astounding. After the first month, we stopped synchronizing our eating, and started relying more on our innate knowledge of the program in order to be successful. Dave ended up loving the 20:4 fasting days, and by the end of the second month, Dave was down another 7 kilos! But, the best thing about it was, even after the second month, there still wasn't much of a lifestyle change. None of us were craving anything sugary, nor were we craving any kind of breads. And, we never found ourselves excessively hungry.

That was the best thing about the ketogenic diet, that set it apart it from other weight loss strategies.

The thing Dave likes the best is that there's no calorie counting. Using percentages of fats, proteins, and carbs and working them into accurate ratios to figure out how many grams of each to take in, negates the need to count calories. With a ketogenic diet, the focus isn't on the number of calories you cut out, but on the number of grams of certain macronutrients that you eat.

The emphasis isn't on cutting out, but putting in.

I think that's why none of us really struggled with hunger pains.

One of the tricks Dave adopted was using smaller dinner plates when he was eating. It helped him to further control his portions, and he found that it worked for him. Jared took this much more seriously than we thought he would. In the last few weeks he found different ways to test his ketone levels and fully track how much he was consuming in terms of fat, protein, carbohydrates, and calories. Not only that, but he kept track of his measurements, which is a first for the gym-rat!

The outcome, for Jared, was fantastic. He became super lean and very active. His overall body function and work performance peaked. When he was done with the first two- month period, he stopped focusing on counting and measuring because he started trusting himself a bit more. He still regularly went through intermittent fasts and maintained a basic ketogenic eating system so he would shift into ketosis at least twice a month, and would keep a healthy lifestyle otherwise.

Even I did not revert to old habits. It was easy to see the feel and direct benefits of my new eating regimen. It was easy to maintain the ketogenic lifestyle as well. I would do simple intermittent fasting every once in a while, maybe once every two or three weeks. Aside from that, I kept my carb intake low and definitely never went back to a sugar heavy diet.

Overall, it was truly a fantastic experience. And, while Jared and I did enjoy it very much, it was really Dave who took it to heart. When the third month came along, he began to learn how to optimize his ketosis. In fact, across his entire time experimenting with keto and the months after, even his own tune in his diary entries began to change: he saw the difference being made, and he had met his match.

He had found a diet that didn't feel like a diet.

After the third month, Dave was down yet another 3 kilos. He thinks the decrease in weight loss for the overall month was due to his reduced fasting. More likely, it could be because his body had used most of the fat he had stored up as energy by this point. Also, he couldn't believe his "man-boobs" were gone. He kept bragging about it.

That was something he was very proud of.

The greatest change for Dave, aside from the continued weight loss, was that he felt more confident and relaxed in his day to day eating habits. Because we had created a new way of eating, we started to trust our food decisions more instead of relying on strict protocols and rules in the ketogenic diet. This seems to have made him more confident, which is a really good thing.

Dave was struggling with his confidence up until this point.

Dave also told us that he no longer wanted to get himself down to 65kg. He lost the weight during the third month and thought he looked fantastic, which is something we've never heard him say before. His focus shifted a bit.

After the fourth month, Dave was down to 70kg. He started going to the gym to work on building muscle, and he stuck to his goal of becoming more active, in general. He was still hesitant to talk about the fact that he was on a "diet," and kept calling it a "lifestyle change" more than anything. Jared and I also kept through, mostly, for the four months. All in all, Francis had gone down 16 kilos during the four months and I had gone down 13 kilos, which was really nice. We celebrated our triumphs with a couple of bottles of wine.

One thing we found with our weigh-ins, though, was not to obsess over the numbers. If you get too distracted with the numbers on the scale, you miss the whole point, which is the freedom that the ketogenic diet provides. It really is the most relaxed weight loss system any of us have ever tried. Partly because we didn't have to stress about counting calories or weighing and charting our progress after every week.

With a lifestyle change like this, there are a few things to keep in mind. Results are always going to vary from person to person, just like it did between the two of us. Also, your doctor should always be consulted when making major dietary changes. It is imperative to keep hydrated. This is not just a way to stave of those random cravings, it is also something that's going to help with the dreaded keto adaptation period in the first week.

Make sure everything you cook, is actually cooked at home. As in, don't go out and expect those frozen, pre-packaged meals that advertise themselves as "healthy" to actually be healthy. Stay as far away from those as possible. The best way to know what you're eating isn't loaded with sugar or harmful additives is to actually make it yourself.

Another important thing is that you simply need to eat when you're hungry. Society has taught us that there are designated points during the day where you need to eat, and the rest of the time you don't. That can be really dangerous, especially if the typical "three basic meals" are not getting your body enough nutrients. On the ketogenic diet, simply eat when you get hungry. If you're not hungry for the first two hours after you've woken up, then don't eat. If you get hungry an hour before your lunch break, then take your lunch early or eat a keto-friendly snack. Your body is hungry for a reason. Just give it what it needs when it needs it.

Any diet, including this one, is not a temporary fix. When you make the switch in your eating habits, it's for good. If you stop the ketogenic diet and expect to keep the weight off, you're going to gain the weight back. This is what "yo-yo dieting" is, and it affects hundreds of thousands of people around the world. A slow change in routine is going to help prepare your mind for the change in your lifestyle, and it will increase the likelihood of a ketogenic diet becoming a ketogenic lifestyle.

After you learn how a ketogenic diet works and learn the types of foods you can and can't eat, it becomes very possible for someone to make their own food plan. Greens are always a good thing to work into your diet because of their nutrient and fiber contents. Fat intake has to be prioritized above all else because that is the largest percentage of your macronutrients that you will be taking in.

And, of course, it always helps to do it with someone. The three of us were able to keep each other on track and celebrate with one another when we achieved our goals. This isn't necessary, but it sure helps.

All in all, this is definitely a lifestyle we can do. There's no calorie counting. There's no random cravings for ice cream at 2 AM. There are ways to tweak the diet even if we do decide to go out, and there are still alcohols we can drink while doing it! It's the most enjoyable diet we have found that actually delivers results. At the end of it all, it was a fantastic journey that taught us a lot about the way we eat and what's actually in our food. It was a dietary experience that truly enriched us. Now we look healthy, lean and handsome, just because we wanted to help a friend out.

In order to help you experience the same great lifestyle change, I've created a massive keto recipe book with 100 awesome menu options. Feel free to use your own creativity in the kitchen as well. Eating keto is healthy, but it should also be delicious. I'd recommend making a big mug of Bulletproof coffee, heading to the kitchen, and beginning a keto journey of your own!

100 Ketogenic Recipes

Part 1: Keto Breakfast Recipes
1) Mushroom, Eggs and Avocado Breakfast

Serves: 2

Ingredients:

- 1 medium avocado, peeled, pitted, sliced
- 3 eggs
- 5 large Portobello mushrooms
- 8 bacon slices
- 3 tablespoons butter or ghee
- Salt and pepper as per taste
- Fresh herbs of your choice to garnish

Method:

1. Place a nonstick skillet over medium low heat. Add half the butter.
2. Place the mushrooms with its topside down. Season with salt and pepper and cook until mushrooms are tender.
3. Remove from the pan and place on a serving platter.
4. Place the pan back on heat and add the remaining butter. Add bacon. Crack the eggs in it and cook until done.
5. Remove on to the serving platter.
6. Serve with avocado slices.

2) Cream Cheese Pancakes

Serves: 4

Ingredients

- 2 oz. cream cheese
- 2 large eggs
- 1 tablespoon sugar substitute
- 1 tablespoon rolled oats
- ½ teaspoon cinnamon
- Some strawberries for garnish

Method:

1. In a large bowl, beat some cream cheese using a spoon or an electric beater until it is nice and fluffy.
2. Now crack the eggs, one by one and beat the mixture again.
3. Lightly crush the oats using a pounder.
4. Drizzle some sugar substitute, cinnamon powder and gently fold it in.
5. Grease a saucepan with some oil or butter and heat it over medium flame.
6. Add one scoop of batter and gently spread it across the pan. Cook the pancake for about 2 minutes until they turn golden brown. Now flip it over and cook for another minute. Repeat the process for the remaining batter.
7. Transfer to a large dish.
8. Roughly chop some strawberries and add them on top of the pancakes.
9. Serve warm.

3) Spicy Granola Bake

Serves: 4

Ingredients

- 1 cup pecans, chopped
- ½ cup walnuts, chopped
- ½ cup almonds, slivered
- ½ cup coconut flakes, unsweetened
- ½ cup almond meal
- ¼ cup flax meal
- ¼ cup pepitas
- ¼ cup sunflower seeds
- ¼ cup melted butter
- ½ cup sugar substitute
- 1 tablespoon honey
- 1 teaspoon cinnamon powder
- 1 teaspoon vanilla
- ½ teaspoon nutmeg
- ½ teaspoon salt
- ¼ cup water

Method:

1. Preheat the oven to 330 F.
2. In a large bowl, combine all the nuts with flax meal, pepitas, sunflower seeds, sugar substitute, honey, ground cinnamon, nutmeg, salt, almond meal, coconut flakes and mix well using a spoon.
3. Drizzle some melted butter on top along with some almond meal and gently fold it in.
4. Place a parchment paper on a baking tray.
5. Transfer the granola tray and place another sheet of parchment paper on the granola. Now firm it using a rolling pin and even it out.
6. Place the tray in the oven and bake it for up to 90 minutes until brown and crisp. Let it cool off for about 30 minutes and store in an airtight container.
7. You can mix some granola with chilled almond milk and eat it for breakfast.

4) Egg White Frittata

Serves: 1

Ingredients:

- 4 egg whites
- 1 cup fresh spinach
- 1 small onion, chopped
- 1 small green bell pepper
- 1 small red bell pepper
- 1/4 cup feta cheese, crumbled
- 1 tablespoon olive oil
- 1/2 teaspoon kosher salt or to taste
- 1/2 teaspoon black pepper powder

Method:

1. Place a heavy ovenproof skillet over medium low heat. Add oil. When oil is heated, add onion and bell peppers and sauté until tender.
2. Season with salt and pepper.
3. Add egg whites and cook for about 3 minutes.
4. Sprinkle spinach and cheese over the egg whites.
5. Transfer the skillet into a preheated oven and bake at 375-degree F for 8-10 minutes.
6. When done, run the edges with a knife and invert over a serving plate.
7. Serve hot.

5) Ketogenic Pancakes

Serves: 6

Ingredients:

- 1 1/2 cups almond meal
- 6 tablespoons almond milk, unsweetened or more if required
- 2 small eggs
- 1/2 tablespoon ground flaxseed
- 1/4 teaspoon baking soda
- 1/4 teaspoon sea salt
- 1 tablespoon coconut oil or butter melted + extra for greasing the pan

Method:

1. Whisk together eggs and milk in a large bowl. Add oil or butter and whisk again until well blended.
2. Mix together all the dry ingredients in a bowl and add to the egg mixture little by little, whisking each time.
3. Add more milk if you find the batter too thick. Add a tablespoon at a time and whisk.
4. Place a nonstick skillet over medium heat. Grease the pan lightly. Pour about 1/4 cup batter on the pan. Slightly swirl the pan so that the batter spreads a little. Slowly bubbles will form and the edges will begin to cook.
5. Cook until the underside is golden brown. Flip sides and cook the other side too.
6. Repeat steps 4-5 with the remaining batter. It makes about 6-7 pancakes
7. Serve with yogurt and fresh fruits.

6) Raspberry Pancakes

Serves: 1

Ingredients:

- 1 banana
- 4 tablespoons almond milk
- 1 ½ cups frozen raspberries
- ½ cup egg whites
- 4 tablespoons Greek yogurt
- 2 tablespoons Chia seeds
- 2 scoops Protein powder
- 2 tablespoons Cinnamon

Method:

1. Peel the banana and mash it finely.
2. Take the chia seeds and grind it into a nice powder.
3. Take a small bowl. Add the protein powder, almond milk, egg whites, and mashed banana, ground chia, cinnamon to the bowl and mix them well.
4. Once it becomes a fine mixture, toss in the frozen raspberries. Stir well.
5. Pour the batter on a slightly heated pan. Cook the pancakes over medium heat. Once the edges of the pancake turn brown, flip it and cook the other side.
6. Transfer the cooked pancakes to a clean plate. Serve it with the Greek yogurt.

7) Fish and Egg Breakfast Bowl

Serves: 2

Ingredients:

- 4 thin slices wild smoked salmon
- 4 eggs
- 1/2 avocado, diced
- 1 cup arugula
- 2 teaspoons ghee
- Lemon juice as required
- Freshly ground black pepper
- Salt to taste

Method:

1. Place a nonstick pan over medium heat. Add ghee and cook the eggs, sunny side up.
2. Meanwhile, divide and arrange arugula, avocado and smoked salmon in 2 serving bowls.
3. Sprinkle salt, pepper and lemon juice over it. When the eggs are done, gently slice the eggs and place in the bowl.
4. Serve immediately.

8) Grain Free Cauliflower Hash Browns

Serves: 2

Ingredients

- 1 large head of cauliflower, approximately 1 lb.
- 1 large egg
- ¼ teaspoon salt
- ¼ teaspoon ground black pepper
- 1 tablespoon finely chopped onion
- 1 tablespoon finely chopped red bell pepper
- 1 tablespoon finely chopped green bell pepper
- 2 tablespoons cottage cheese
- 1 teaspoon olive oil

Method:

1. Wash the cauliflower properly and pat it dry. Now rice it using a grater. Set aside.
2. In a bowl, crack the eggs and beat them lightly. To this, add the cauliflower rice, some peppers, onion, salt, ground black pepper, and whisk well until nice and smooth.
3. Heat a saucepan over medium flame. Add some olive oil and spread it across the pan.
4. Add half of the cauliflower mix and spread it across the pan using a spatula.
5. Now let the hash brown cook for about 4-5 minutes until it starts turning golden brown and then flip it over.
6. Add some more onions and cottage cheese on top of the hash brown.
7. Let the hash brown cook until the cheese has slightly melted. Repeat the process with the remaining batter.
8. Serve warm.

9) Cheesy Quinoa Egg Bake

Serves: 3

Ingredients:

- 4 eggs
- 1/4 cup quinoa, uncooked, rinsed, drained
- 10 tablespoons nonfat milk
- 1 cup packed baby spinach, roughly chopped
- 1 teaspoon butter
- 1 teaspoon garlic, minced
- 1/2 cup Romano or parmesan cheese, chopped
- 1 teaspoon thyme, chopped
- 1/4 teaspoon salt
- 1/4 teaspoon pepper powder

Method:

1. Whisk together in a bowl, eggs, milk, garlic, thyme, and pepper powder and salt.
2. Add quinoa and whisk again.
3. Add spinach and stir.
4. Pour into a butter greased baking dish. Cover the dish with aluminum foil. Tilt the dish gently so that the quinoa spreads well at the bottom of the dish.
5. Bake in a preheated oven at 350-degree F for about 45 minutes or until set.
6. Uncover and sprinkle cheese all over the top.
7. Bake for another 15 minutes or until the top is golden brown.
8. Remove from oven and let it cool for a while.
9. Slice and serve immediately.

10) Special Breakfast Meatloaf

Serves: 4

Ingredients

- 1 teaspoon ghee or butter
- 6 large eggs
- 1 lb. Italian sausage
- ¼ yellow onion, finely chopped
- 1 cup cheddar cheese, grated
- 2 tablespoons scallion

Method:

1. Preheat the oven to 350 F.
2. Grease a baking pan using some cooking spray and set aside.
3. Place the sausages on a cutting board and chop them up it thick slices using a sharp knife.
4. In a bowl, crack the eggs and beat them lightly using a fork. Now add the sausage pieces, onion, and some cream cheese and whisk thoroughly.
5. Pour this batter into the baking tray and set it in the oven.
6. Bake for 30 minutes uncovered until it is golden brown.
7. Remove the dish from the oven and let it cool off for 5 minutes.
8. Now take the remaining cream cheese and spread it across the meatloaf. Add some grated cheese on top along with the scallions.
9. Place the tray in the oven and bake again for 5 minutes. Now broil it for 2-3 minutes until the cheese starts turning golden and crisp.
10. Serve warm.

11) Eggs with Italian Baked Veggies

Serves: 2

Ingredients:

- 1/2 zucchini, quartered lengthwise, chopped crosswise into 3/4 inch pieces
- 1/2 red bell pepper, chopped into 3/4 inch pieces
- 1/2 pound plum tomatoes, chopped into 1 inch chunks
- 1 large clove garlic, minced
- 1 small onion, halved, sliced
- 2 tablespoon fat free parmesan cheese
- 2 large eggs
- Salt to taste
- Pepper powder to taste
- 1/2 teaspoon dried basil
- Cooking spray

Method:

1. Spray a roasting pan with cooking spray. Place tomatoes, zucchini, onion, bell pepper, basil and garlic in the roasting pan.
2. Season with salt and pepper. Spray a little cooking spray. Toss well.
3. Roast in a preheated oven at 400-degree F for about 30 minutes or until the vegetables are tender and brown.
4. Grease 2 ramekins or custard cups with cooking spray. Divide and place the vegetables in the cup.
5. Make a cavity in the center of the vegetables and crack an egg into each of the cavity in the cups.
6. Sprinkle cheese over it. Place the filled cups on a baking sheet. Bake at 400-degree F for 20-25 minutes or until the eggs are set.

12) Turkey Breakfast Sausages

Serves: 3

Ingredients:

- 1 pound extra lean ground turkey breast
- 1/4 teaspoon cayenne pepper or to taste
- 1/2 teaspoon ground ginger
- 1/2 teaspoon sage
- 1/2 teaspoon salt or to taste
- 1/8 teaspoon pepper powder
- Cooking spray

Method:

1. Add cayenne pepper, ginger, sage, salt and pepper to a bowl and mix well.
2. Add turkey and mix well using your hands until the mixture is well combined.
3. Divide the mixture into 6 portions and shape into patties.
4. Place a nonstick pan over medium heat. Spray with cooking spray.
5. Place the patties on the pan and cook until the underside is brown. Flip sides and cook the other side too. The center of the patties should not be pink.
6. Serve hot.

13) Oriental Breakfast Scramble

Serves: 2

Ingredients:

- 2 tablespoons scallion, sliced
- 2 teaspoons fresh ginger, peeled, minced
- 4 teaspoon coconut oil or ghee
- 4 small garlic cloves, minced
- 6 eggs, well beaten
- 1 teaspoon chili powder
- A large pinch freshly ground black pepper
- 2 tablespoon fresh cilantro, chopped
- Salt to taste

Method:

1. Place a medium skillet over medium high heat. Add coconut oil. When oil is heated, add ginger, garlic, and scallions.
2. Stir-fry for a few seconds until fragrant and add beaten eggs. Scramble the eggs by stirring constantly and cook until done.
3. Sprinkle salt, chili powder, and pepper powder.
4. Add cilantro. Mix well.
5. Remove from heat and serve.

14) Roasted Vegetables and Eggs

Serves: 2

Ingredients:

- 1 large head cauliflower, cut into medium sized florets
- 4 small heads broccoli, cut into medium sized florets
- 2 eggs
- 1 teaspoon red pepper flakes
- 1/2 teaspoon salt
- 1/2 teaspoon pepper powder
- 1/2 teaspoon garlic powder
- 3 tablespoons extra virgin olive oil + extra for cooking eggs
- Juice of a lemon
- Hot sauce to taste

Method:

1. Add cauliflower and broccoli to a large bowl. Add oil and toss. Add garlic powder salt, pepper and red pepper flakes and toss again.
2. Transfer on to a baking sheet. Sprinkle lemon juice all over the vegetables.
3. Place in a preheated oven and bake at 400-degree F for about 15 minutes.
4. Meanwhile, place a nonstick pan over medium heat. Add a little olive oil over it and swirl the pan.
5. Crack the eggs in the pan and cook until the underside is done. Flip sides and cook the other side for 20-30 seconds. Remove the eggs and place an egg each over 2 serving plates.
6. Divide the vegetables and place along with the eggs. Sprinkle some more red pepper flakes, add a dash of hot sauce and serve.

15) Cauliflower Hash Cajun Style

Serves: 2

Ingredients:

- 2 tablespoons olive oil
- 1 small onion, diced into 4 pieces
- 2 tablespoons minced garlic
- 1 lb. cauliflower florets
- 1 tablespoon Cajun seasoning
- 8 oz. red pastrami, shaved
- 1 small green bell pepper, diced into 4 pieces

Method:

1. Heat some olive oil or ghee in a saucepan over medium flame.
2. Add some minced garlic, chopped onions and sauté them for about 3-4 minutes until they turn golden brown.
3. Boil some water in a vessel and add the cauliflower florets in it Remove from flame and cover with a lid for 5 minutes. Once done, drain the water and add some cold water to the vessel. Now drain off the cold water too and using your hands, squeeze out all the excess water from the cauliflower florets.
4. Add the florets to the saucepan and fry for 10 minutes until it starts to brown.
5. Add some Cajun seasoning and toss all the ingredients well.
6. Slide in the chopped peppers and pastrami and mix. Cook for 5 minutes and remove from flame.
7. Transfer the mixture into a large bowl.
8. Fry an egg over the saucepan and place it on top.
9. Sprinkle some more Cajun seasoning and serve.

16) Ham and Eggs

Serves: 3

Ingredients:

- 6 slices ham, preservative free
- 6 eggs
- 1/2 teaspoon paprika
- 1/2 teaspoon pepper powder or to taste
- Salt to taste

Method:

1. Take a muffin tin and line the muffin cups with slices of ham.
2. Break an egg into each of the muffin cups.
3. Sprinkle, salt, paprika and pepper over the eggs.
4. Bake in a preheated oven at 375-degree F for about 20 minutes or until eggs are set.
5. Remove from oven and cool for a few minutes.
6. Loosen the edges with a knife and remove the muffins and serve.

17) Breakfast Skillet

Serves: 2

Ingredients:

- 6 egg whites
- 6 slices turkey bacon, cut into 1/2 inch pieces
- 1 tablespoon olive oil
- 1/4 cup red bell pepper, chopped
- 1/4 cup green bell pepper, chopped
- 1/2 cup onions, chopped
- 1/2 cup part skim mozzarella cheese
- 1/4 teaspoon garlic powder
- 1/4 teaspoon pepper powder or to taste
- Salt to taste

Method:

1. Place a skillet over medium heat. Add bell peppers, onion, garlic powder and bacon.
2. Sauté until the bacon is brown and the vegetables are slightly soft,
3. Add egg whites and keep stirring until the eggs are cooked through.
4. Add cheese and mix Season with salt and pepper. Mix well and serve.

18) Ketogenic Tomato Frittata

Serves: 4

Ingredients:

- 1 medium onion, halved, sliced
- 12 large eggs
- 1 1/3 cups cherry tomatoes, halved
- 1/4 cup fresh basil or chives, chopped
- 1 1/3 cup feta cheese, crumbled
- Salt to taste
- Freshly ground black pepper to taste
- 2 tablespoons ghee

Method:

1. Place an ovenproof skillet over medium heat. Add ghee. When melts, add onions and sauté until brown.
2. Meanwhile whisk together eggs with salt and pepper. Add herbs and whisk again.
3. Pour eggs over the onions. Do not stir and cook until the edges begin to cook. Remove the skillet from heat.
4. Sprinkle tomatoes over it followed by cheese.
5. Place the skillet in a preheated oven and broil at 400-degree F until the top is golden brown.
6. Remove from heat and cool for a while. Divide into 4 wedges and serve

19) Chocolate Hazelnut Waffles

Serves: 12

Ingredients:

- 2 cups hazelnut meal
- 1/4 cup coconut flour
- 1/4 cup cocoa powder
- 8 large eggs
- 6 tablespoons hazelnut oil
- 6 tablespoons stevia sweetener or granulated xylitol
- 1/2 teaspoon stevia extract
- 1 cup chocolate protein powder
- 2/3 cup full fat Greek yogurt
- 1/2 teaspoon stevia extract
- A little melted ghee for greasing

Method:

1. Add hazelnut meal, chocolate protein powder, cocoa powder, coconut flour and sweetener to a large bowl and mix well.
2. Add eggs, yogurt, hazelnut oil, hazelnut extract and stevia and whisk well to get a smooth batter.
3. Preheat a waffle iron to medium high. Grease the waffle iron with ghee. Pour about 1/4 cup of batter into each of the waffle mold.
4. Gently close the lid and cook until crisp and brown.
5. Remove the waffles and place on a baking sheet in an oven to keep warm.
6. Make more waffles with the remaining batter.
7. This batter makes about 12 waffles.
8. Serve with a topping of your choice like berries, whipped cream, etc.
   Note: Nutritional value of topping is not included in the above-mentioned values

20) Keto Pumpkin Bagels

Serves: Makes 16 bagels

Ingredients:

- 6 eggs, beaten
- 6 tablespoons golden flax meal
- 1 cup coconut flour, sifted
- 1/2 cup coconut milk or almond milk, unsweetened
- 4 tablespoons coconut oil or butter, melted + extra for greasing
- 2 1/2 teaspoons pumpkin pie spice
- 1 cup pumpkin puree
- 1 teaspoon ground cinnamon
- 3 teaspoons xylitol
- 30 drops stevia
- 1 teaspoon baking soda
- 2 teaspoons apple cider vinegar
- 1/4 teaspoon sea salt
- 1 teaspoon vanilla extract

Method:

1. Mix together in a large bowl, coconut flour, flax meal, pumpkin pie spice, cinnamon and sea salt and set aside.
2. Whisk together eggs, pumpkin puree, milk, vanilla extract, butter, xylitol, and stevia in a bowl.
3. Mix together baking soda and vinegar in a bowl and add to the egg mixture. Mix well.
4. Pour this mixture into the coconut flour mixture and whisk until a smooth batter is formed.
5. Grease bagel pans with oil or butter. Carefully pour the batter into the pans. Ensure that the hole part of the pan is clean without any batter dropped over it. If so, wipe with a moist paper towel.
6. Bake in a preheated oven at 350-degree F for about 23-25 minutes.
7. Remove the pans from the oven and let it cool.
8. Gently loosen the edges with a knife and remove the bagels from the mold.
9. Serve with desired topping of your choice.

Part 2: Ketogenic Breakfast Smoothies

21) Green Goddess

Serves: 2

Ingredients:

- 3 cups fresh spinach
- 1 ripe avocado, peeled, pitted, chopped into pieces
- 1 ½ cup almond milk, unsweetened
- 2 scoops whey protein powder
- 1/2 teaspoon peppermint extract
- 8 drops stevia or as per taste
- Ice as required

Method:

1. Add all the ingredients to a blender and blend until smooth.
2. Pour into tall glasses and serve.

22) Avocado Spinach Smoothie

Serves: 2
Ingredients:

- 1 avocado
- 1/2 cup coconut milk
- 1/2 cup spinach leaves (chopped)
- 1/2 cup fresh mint leaves
- 1 ½ scoop whey powder, vanilla flavored
- 2 tablespoons powdered pistachio
- 1 teaspoon vanilla essence
- 6 drops liquid stevia
- 1/2 cup water
- 3 ice cubes

Method:

1. Chop the avocado coarsely and add it to a blender.
2. Pour coconut milk and chopped spinach leaves. Add half a cup of fresh mint leaves as well.
3. Add one scoop of vanilla flavored whey protein powder to the mixture.
4. Add 2 tablespoons of pistachio powder. Blend it all for about a minute
5. To this mixture add a teaspoon of vanilla extract and 6 drops of liquid stevia.
6. Pour water and add the ice cubes.
7. Blend at medium speed for 2 minutes until smooth.
8. Serve chilled immediately.

23) Weight Loss Smoothie

Serves: 2

Ingredients:

- 2 cups water
- 1 medium avocado
- 1 cup fresh or frozen blueberries
- 2 tablespoons chia seeds or chia seed gel
- 1 tablespoon coconut oil
- ½ teaspoon ground cinnamon
- 1 tablespoon honey or stevia or maple syrup
- Ice cubes

Method:

1. Add all the ingredients to a blender and blend until smooth.
2. Pour into tall glasses and serve immediately.

24) Strawberry with Coconut Milk

Serves: 4

Ingredients:
- 2 cups coconut milk, unsweetened
- 2 cups strawberries, frozen
- 4 tablespoons smooth almond butter
- Few drops stevia to taste (optional)

Method:
1. Add all the ingredients to a blender and blend until smooth.
2. Pour into tall glasses and serve.

25) Green Tea Kiwi Smoothie

Serves: 2

Ingredients:

- 2 medium kiwi fruits
- 1 1/2 cups freshly brewed green tea
- 1/4 cup lemon juice
- 1 cup lettuce leaves, torn

Method:

1. Add all the ingredients to the blender and blend for about 20-30 seconds or until smooth.
2. Pour into a tall glass and serve with crushed ice.

26) Chocolaty Berry Protein Smoothie

Serves: 2

Ingredients

- 2 cups coconut milk, unsweetened
- 1 cup fresh cherries, pitted (If using frozen, thawed)
- 2/3 cup hemp hearts
- 2 scoops protein powder
- 1/2 cup cocoa powder, unsweetened
- 1 teaspoon liquid chocolate stevia
- Ice as required

Method:

1. Add all the ingredients to a blender and blend until smooth.
2. Pour into tall glasses and serve.

27) Minty Green Smoothie

Serves: 1

Ingredients:

- 1 cup tall kale
- 1 small avocado, peeled, pitted, chopped
- 2 teaspoons chlorella
- 1 cup mint leaves
- 2 tablespoons lemon juice
- 2 tablespoons lime juice
- 1 1/2 cups water
- Ice as required

Method:

1. Add all the ingredients to the blender and blend until smooth.
2. Pour into tall glasses and serve immediately.

28) Coconut Milk and Avocado Smoothie

Serves: 2
Ingredients:

- 2 avocados
- 1/2-cup coconut milk.
- 1/2 cup kiwis
- 1 scoop whey powder, vanilla flavored
- 1 tablespoon chia seeds
- 6 drops liquid stevia
- 1/2 cup water
- 3 ice cubes
- Cinnamon Powder (for garnish, optional)

Method:

1. Scoop the avocados and keep aside.
2. Add the avocados and half a cup of coconut milk to a blender.
3. Add half a cup of freshly cut kiwis to the mixture and 1 scoop of vanilla flavored whey protein powder. Blend for 30 seconds on medium.
4. Add the chia seeds and liquid stevia to the mixture in the blender.
5. Pour half a cup of water and ice cubes into the blender.
6. Blend at medium speed until smooth.
7. Garnish with cinnamon powder and serve chilled.

29) Flax Seed and Blueberry

Serves: 2

Ingredients:

- 2 cups spinach (fresh)
- 1 cup almond milk
- 1 cup blueberries (frozen)
- 2 papayas (frozen)
- 2 tbsp. ground flax seed

Method:

- Place the ingredients in the blender and blend for one minute or till the mixture is smooth.
- Pour it into a glass and serve immediately. Add ice to the top of the glass and serve.

30) Cinnamon Smoothie

Serves: 2

Ingredients:

- 2 cups almond milk
- 1 teaspoon cinnamon powder
- 4 tablespoons vanilla protein powder
- 2 teaspoons flax meal
- 1/2 teaspoon vanilla extract
- Stevia drops to taste
- Ice as required

Method:

1. Add all the ingredients to a blender and blend until smooth.
2. Pour into tall glasses and serve.

31) Pina Colada

Serves: 2

Ingredients:

- 1 cup almond milk (unsweetened preferably)
- 1 cup coconut water
- 1 cup pineapple (frozen)
- 2 tsp. honey
- 1 tbsp. shredded coconut
- ½ tsp. vanilla extract

Method:

- Place the ingredients in the blender and blend for one minute or till the mixture is smooth.
- Pour it into a glass and serve immediately. Add ice to the top of the glass and serve.

32) Creamy Egg Breakfast Shake

Serves: 2

Ingredients:

- 4 large eggs
- 8-10 drops stevia or to taste
- 1/2 cup full fat coconut milk
- 2 scoops chocolate- greens powder
- Banana Capella flavor drops to taste
- Ice cubes as required

Method:

1. Add all the ingredients to a blender and blend until smooth.
2. Pour into tall glasses and serve.

33) Blackberry Smoothie

Serves: 2

Ingredients

- 1 cup blackberries, fresh or frozen
- 1/2 cup heavy whipping cream
- 1/2 cup full fat cream cheese or creamed coconut milk
- 2 tablespoons extra virgin coconut oil
- 1 cup water
- 1 teaspoon vanilla extract
- 5-7 drops stevia (optional)

Method:

1. Add all the ingredients to a blender and blend until smooth.
2. Pour into tall glasses and serve.

34) Fat Bomb Smoothie

Serves: 2

Ingredients:

- 3 cups coconut milk
- 3 cups heavy cream
- 1/4 cup unrefined coconut oil
- 3 cups strawberries
- A pinch of salt

Method:

1. Place all the ingredients in a blender and blend until smooth.
2. Pour into tall glasses.
3. Serve immediately with crushed ice.

35) Butter Bomb smoothie

Serves: 2

Ingredients:

- 2 cups almond milk
- 2 papayas
- 1 tbsp. roasted chia seeds
- 3 tbsp. peanut butter
- ½ tsp. vanilla essence

Method:

- Place the ingredients in the blender and blend for one minute or till the mixture is smooth.
- Pour it into a glass and serve immediately. Add ice to the top of the glass and serve.

36) Spicy Strawberry Smoothie

Serves: 2

Ingredients:

- 1 pound strawberries, hulled (unsweetened if frozen)
- 1 medium cucumber, peeled, coarsely chopped
- 2 small Roma tomatoes
- 1 cup light coconut milk
- Juice of 2 limes
- 1 cup ice
- 1/2 teaspoon ground cayenne pepper + extra to garnish
- Honey to taste
- A pinch of salt
- Lime slices to garnish
- Strawberries to garnish

Method:

1. Add all the ingredients to a blender and blend until smooth.
2. Pour into tall glasses. Sprinkle some cayenne pepper. Garnish with strawberries and lime slices. Serve immediately.

37) Chocolate and Almond Smoothie

Serves: 2

Ingredients:

- 2 scoops chocolate whey protein
- 2 cups coconut milk
- 2 tbsp. roasted almond
- 1 tbsp. grated coconut
- 1 tsp. almond extract

Method:

- Place the ingredients in the blender and blend for one minute or till the mixture is smooth.
- Pour it into a glass and serve immediately. Add ice to the top of the glass and serve.

38) Heart Healthy Smoothie

Serves: 2

Ingredients:

- ½ cup walnuts
- 2 tbsp. cinnamon
- 2 tsp. ginger
- 2 tsp. nutmeg
- 2 tbsp. almond butter
- 2 mashed papayas
- 3 whole eggs
- ½ cup almond milk
- 1 cup mixed berries

Method:

- Blend the spices and nuts in a food processer till you obtain a grain like consistency and set aside.
- Whisk the milk and eggs together and blend the mixture with the almond butter and mashed papaya.
- Add the spice and nut mixture and warm till you obtain the desired consistency.
- Store in the refrigerator. Serve with crushed ice.

39) Berry Blast Smoothie

Serves: 2

Ingredients:

- 1 cup strawberries (hulled)
- 1 cup blueberries
- 1 cup plain yoghurt
- 1 cup milk
- 1 tbsp. vanilla protein powder

Method:

- Place the ingredients in the blender and blend for one minute or till the mixture is smooth.
- Pour it into a glass and serve immediately. You can add crushed ice to the top of the glass and serve to keep the smoothie cold.

40) Chocolate Smoothie

Serves: 2

Ingredients:

- 8-ounce almond milk, unsweetened
- Few drops stevia or any other artificial sweetener to taste
- 3 ounces heavy cream
- 1 scoop chocolate flavored whey powder
- Crushed ice to serve (optional)

Method:

1. Place all the ingredients in a blender and blend until smooth.
2. Pour into tall glasses. Serve with crushed ice.

Part 3: Ketogenic Salad, Soups and Stew Recipes

41) Crunchy and Nutty Cauliflower Salad

Serves: 6

Ingredients:

- 6 cups cauliflower, very finely chopped
- 1 cup walnuts, chopped
- 2 cups leeks, green parts only, finely chopped
- Unrefined sea salt to taste
- Freshly ground pepper to taste
- 2 cups sour cream

Method:

1. Add all the ingredients in a large bowl. Toss well. Cover and chill for 3-4 hours for the flavors to set in.
2. Serve cold.

42) Tricolor Salad

Serves: 4

Ingredients:

- 7-8 medium tomatoes, sliced
- ¼ cup extra virgin olive oil
- 1 cup mozzarella di bufala or mozzarella for salads, cubed
- 2 large avocadoes, pitted, peeled, sliced
- 10 kalamata olives, sliced
- ¼ cup pesto
- Salt to taste
- Pepper powder to taste
- 2 tablespoons fresh basil, chopped

Method:

1. Add all the ingredients to a large bowl. Toss well and serve right away.

43) Chicken Salad Wraps

Serves: 4-6
Ingredients:
For chicken:

- 2 pounds chicken thighs
- 1 teaspoon salt or to taste
- 1 teaspoon pepper powder or to taste
- 2 tablespoons olive oil
- ½ teaspoon garlic powder

For salad:

- 2 cups celery, diced
- 1 cup keto friendly mayonnaise
- Pepper to taste
- Salt to taste
- 20 Baby Cos lettuce or Romaine lettuce leaves
- 2 tablespoons fresh parsley, finely chopped

Method:
1. To make chicken: Add chicken, pepper, salt, oil and garlic powder into a bowl. Toss well.
2. Transfer the chicken on to a lined baking sheet.
3. Roast in a preheated oven at 390° F for 20-30 minutes or until done.
4. When done, remove from the oven and place on your cutting board. When cool enough to handle, chop into small cubes of about 1 centimeter.
5. Add the chopped chicken into a bowl. Add celery, parsley, salt and pepper.
6. Add mayonnaise and fold gently. Taste and adjust the seasonings and mayonnaise if necessary.
7. Place lettuce leaves on a serving platter. Divide the salad over the lettuce leaves.
8. Serve.

44) Mixed Green Spring Salad with Raspberry Vinaigrette

Serves: 4

Ingredients:

- 8 ounces mixed greens
- ½ cup parmesan cheese, shaved
- 1/3 cup pine nuts, roasted
- Pepper to taste
- Salt to taste
- 8 slices bacon

For the keto raspberry vinaigrette dressing:

- 2 tablespoons white vinegar
- 8-9 drops liquid stevia
- 2 tablespoons extra virgin olive oil
- 2 tablespoons golden raspberries

Method:

1. To make the dressing: Add all the ingredients of the dressing into a blender and blend until smooth. Alternately blend with an immersion blender. Transfer into a bowl. Cover and set aside for a while for the flavors to set in.
2. Place a nonstick pan over medium heat. Add bacon. Cook until crisp.
3. Remove bacon with a slotted spoon. When cool enough to handle, crumble the bacon.
4. Add rest of the ingredients of the salad into a bowl. Add bacon. Pour as much dressing as required on top and toss well. Taste and adjust the dressing if required.
5. Serve right away.

45) Lemon Poppy Tahini Salad Boats

Serves: 2

Ingredients:

For the salad:

- 8 lettuce leaves or 2 avocados, peeled, pitted, halved
- ½ cup sunflower seeds or ¼ cup tahini
- 1 cup purple cabbage or carrots, shredded

For the dressing:

- 2 tablespoons lemon juice
- 2 tablespoons extra virgin olive oil
- ½ teaspoon ginger, grated or ground ginger
- ½ tablespoon poppy seeds
- 1/8 teaspoon salt
- Pepper to taste

Method:

1. Whisk together all the ingredients of the dressing in a bowl. Set aside for a while for the flavors to set in.
2. Mix together in a bowl, cabbage, sunflower seeds and dressing.
3. Place lettuce leaves or avocado boats on a serving platter. Place the cabbage mixture on the lettuce leaves or in the cavity of the avocadoes and serve.

46) Balsamic Flat Iron Steak Salad

Serves: 2

Ingredients:

- ¾ pound flat iron steak, cut into ½ inch thick slices
- 1 ½ tablespoons avocado oil or olive oil
- 2 ounces cremini mushrooms, sliced
- 1 medium head romaine lettuce, chopped
- ½ red bell pepper, sliced
- ½ orange bell pepper, sliced
- ½ teaspoon garlic salt
- ½ teaspoon Italian seasoning
- ½ teaspoon onion powder
- ½ teaspoon red pepper flakes
- 2 tablespoons balsamic vinegar
- 3 ounces sweet onion, sliced
- 1 clove garlic minced
- 1 small avocado, peeled, pitted, sliced
- 1.5 ounces sun dried tomatoes

Method:

1. Place meat in a bowl. Drizzle vinegar on it. Toss until well combined. Set aside for a while to marinate.
2. Place a skillet over medium low heat. Add oil. When the oil is heated, add mushrooms, garlic, salt, pepper and onion and sauté for 15-20 minutes until golden brown. Remove from heat and set aside.
3. Add romaine, bell peppers, avocado and sun-dried tomatoes into a bowl.
4. Place meat strips in a broiling pan. Do not overlap and place in one layer. Broil in batches if required.
5. Add garlic salt, seasoning, onion powder ad red pepper flakes into a small bowl. Mix well. Sprinkle it over the meat.
6. Place the broiling pan on the top rack and broil for 4-5 minutes for medium rare.
7. Remove from the oven.
8. To assemble: Divide the salad on individual serving plates. Place mushroom mixture on it. Finally place flat iron steak strips and serve.

47) Spinach and Apple Salad

Serves: 2
Ingredients:
For salad:

- 7-8 cups baby spinach leaves, washed
- ½ cup blue cheese, crumbled
- 1 cup red onions, thinly sliced
- 1 small apple, cored, cut into cubes

For feta vinaigrette dressing:

- 6 tablespoons cold pressed olive oil
- 1 clove garlic, finely minced
- 2 slices thin bacon, cooked, crumbled
- 2 ½ tablespoons red wine vinegar
- 1 ounce feta cheese or blue cheese, finely crumbled

Method:
1. To make dressing: Add oil, vinegar, garlic and feta into a blender and blend until smooth. Transfer into a glass bowl. Add bacon and stir. Set aside for a while for the flavors to set in.
2. Spread the spinach leaves on a serving platter.
3. Layer with onions, followed by the apple and finally the cheese.
4. Drizzle as much dressing as required. Toss. Taste and adjust the dressing if required and serve.
5. Store the remaining dressing in an airtight container in the refrigerator. It can last for 2-3 days.

48) Super Simple Tuna Salad

Serves: 2

Ingredients:

- 4 cups mixed greens
- ½ cup fresh parsley, chopped
- 20 large Kalamata olives, pitted
- 1 avocado, peeled, pitted, diced
- 2 cans light tuna chunks in water, drained
- 2 large tomatoes, diced
- ½ cup fresh mint, chopped
- 2 small zucchinis, sliced lengthwise
- 2 green onions, sliced
- 2 tablespoons balsamic vinegar
- 1 ½ teaspoons freshly cracked black pepper or to taste
- 2 tablespoons extra-virgin olive oil
- ½ teaspoon Himalayan or fine sea salt or to taste

Method:

1. Preheat a grill and grill the zucchini slices on both the sides. You can also grill in a grill pan. When cool enough to handle, chop into chunks.
2. Add all the ingredients including the zucchini to a large bowl. Toss gently and serve.

49) Thai BBQ Pork Salad

Serves: 4

Ingredients:

For the salad:

- 20 ounces pork, cooked, pulled (leftover works well)
- ½ cup fresh cilantro, chopped
- 4 cups romaine lettuce
- 1 medium red bell pepper, chopped

For the Thai BBQ sauce:

- 4 tablespoons tomato paste
- 2 teaspoons creamy peanut butter
- Zest of 1 lime, grated
- Juice of 1 lime
- 2 teaspoons red curry paste
- ½ teaspoon red pepper flakes
- 20 drops liquid stevia
- 5-6 tablespoons soy sauce or coconut aminos
- ¼ cup fresh cilantro, chopped
- 2 teaspoons five spice powder
- 3 tablespoons rice wine vinegar
- 2 teaspoons fish sauce
- 1 teaspoon mango extract

Method:

1. To make sauce: Whisk together all the ingredients of the sauce in a bowl and set aside for a while for the flavors to set in.
2. Layer the salad - lettuce, cilantro and red bell pepper in any manner you desire.
3. Place the pork over it. Pour sauce over the pork and serve.

50) Avocado and Egg Salad

Serves: 4

Ingredients:

- 8 large eggs, hardboiled, quartered
- 8 cups mixed lettuce, rinsed
- 4 cloves garlic, crushed
- 2 tablespoons extra virgin olive oil
- 2 large avocadoes, peeled, pitted, sliced
- 1 cup full fat yogurt or ½ cup keto friendly mayonnaise
- 2 teaspoons Dijon mustard
- 2 tablespoons fresh chives
- 2 tablespoons basil, chopped
- 2 tablespoons thyme, chopped
- Salt to taste
- Pepper powder to taste

Method:

1. To make dressing: Whisk together in a bowl yogurt, garlic, Dijon mustard, salt and pepper. Set aside for a while for the flavors to set in.
2. Place salad greens and dressing in a serving bowl and mix well. Layer with avocadoes followed by eggs.
3. Sprinkle chives, basil, thyme, salt and pepper and serve.

51) Kale and Sausage Soup

Serves: 2

Ingredients:

- ½ pound ground sweet Italian sausage
- 1 small carrot, diced
- 1 small onion, chopped
- 1 small head cauliflower, broken into florets
- 2 cloves garlic, crushed
- 2 cups kale, discard hard stems and ribs, chopped
- 2 teaspoons butter
- 1 tablespoon red wine vinegar
- ½ teaspoon dried rubbed sage
- ½ teaspoon dried oregano
- ½ teaspoon crushed red pepper flakes or to taste
- ½ teaspoons dried basil
- 2 cups low sodium chicken broth
- Freshly ground pepper to taste
- Salt to taste
- ½ cup heavy cream

Method:

1. Place a Dutch oven or a soup pot over medium high heat. Add sausage. Cook until brown. Break it simultaneously as it cooks.
2. Remove with a slotted spoon and place on a plate that is lined with paper towels.
3. Discard the fat left behind in the pot.
4. Place the pot over medium heat.
5. Add onion and carrots and sauté until onions are translucent.
6. Add garlic and sauté until fragrant. Add vinegar and scrape the bottom of the pot to remove any brown bits that are stuck.
7. Add spices, herbs, stock and cream and bring to the boil.
8. Add cauliflower and lower the heat. Simmer until cauliflower is tender.
9. Add kale and the sausage. Mix well. Cook until kale wilts. Add salt and pepper and stir.
10. Ladle into soup bowls and serve.

52) Bacon Cheese Burger Soup

Serves: 6

Ingredients:

- 24 ounces ground beef
- 10 slices bacon
- 4 tablespoons butter
- 1 teaspoon garlic powder
- 6 cups beef broth
- 1 teaspoon onion powder
- 3 teaspoons kosher salt or to taste
- 1 teaspoon black pepper powder or to taste
- 4 teaspoons brown mustard
- 5 tablespoons tomato paste
- 2 teaspoons ground cumin
- 1 teaspoon red chili flakes
- 2 medium pickled dill, diced
- 6 ounces cream cheese
- 2 cups cheddar cheese, shredded
- 1 cup heavy cream

Method:

1. Place a large nonstick pan over medium heat. Place a few bacon slices and cook until brown on both the sides. Remove with a slotted spoon and place on paper towels. Cook the rest in batches. When cool enough to handle, crumble the bacon.
2. To the same pan add beef and cook until brown. Remove with a slotted spoon and set aside.
3. Place a large pot over medium heat. Add butter. When butter melts, add cumin, chili flakes, onion powder, garlic powder, mustard, salt and pepper. Cook for a few seconds and add the beef, broth, tomato paste, pickle and cheddar cheese. Bring to the boil. Add cream cheese. Mix well.
4. Reduce heat, cover with a lid and simmer for about 30-40 minutes. Remove from heat and add cream, crumbled bacon. Mix well.
5. Ladle into soup bowls and serve.

53) Creamy Spinach Soup

Serves: 2

Ingredients:

- 8 cups spinach, chopped
- 4 cloves garlic, sliced
- 1 medium onion, chopped
- ½ cup heavy cream
- 6 tablespoons butter, unsalted
- 1 cup coconut milk, unsweetened
- 2 cups water
- ¼ teaspoon pepper powder
- ¼ teaspoon salt
- 2 tablespoons cream cheese

Method:

1. Place a saucepan over low heat. Add butter. When the butter melts, add garlic and sauté until fragrant. Add onions and sauté until translucent.
2. Add spinach and cook until it wilts.
3. Add water and bring to the boil.
4. Remove from heat and cool for a while. Blend with an immersion blender until smooth.
5. Place the saucepan back on heat. Heat thoroughly
6. Turn off the heat. Add heavy cream and milk and mix.
7. Pour into individual serving bowls.
8. Top with cream cheese and serve.

54) Cream of Chicken Soup with Bacon

Serves: 8

Ingredients:

- 12 slices bacon
- 4 cloves garlic
- 2/3 cup white cooking wine or water
- 1 cup heavy cream
- 8 ribs celery, chopped
- 4 tablespoons butter
- 7 ounces shiitake mushrooms, sliced
- 1 cup coconut milk or almond milk
- 6 cups chicken broth
- 8 pieces chicken thighs, skinless, boneless, cooked, chopped
- Pepper to taste
- Salt to taste
- 4 tablespoons fresh parsley, chopped

Method:

1. Place a large soup pot or Dutch oven over medium heat. Add a little butter and bacon. Cook until crisp. Remove with a slotted spoon and place on paper towels. When cool enough to handle, crumble and set aside for garnishing.
2. Add a little more butter and garlic and sauté until garlic turns golden brown. Add mushrooms and sauté until tender.
3. Add wine and water. Scrape the bottom of the pot to remove any browned bits that are stuck. Simmer until the liquid reduces to half its original quantity.
4. Add rest of the ingredients except parsley. Heat thoroughly.
5. Ladle into soup bowls. Garnish with bacon and serve.

55) Vegan Cream of Mushroom Soup

Serves: 4

Ingredients:

- 4 cups cauliflower florets
- 2 teaspoons onion powder
- 4 cups unsweetened original almond milk
- 2 ½ cups diced white mushrooms
- ½ teaspoon Himalayan rock salt
- Freshly ground pepper to taste
- 1 teaspoon extra-virgin olive oil
- 1 yellow onion, diced

Method:

1. Place a large saucepan over medium heat. Add cauliflower, milk, onion powder, salt and pepper and bring to the boil.
2. Lower heat and cover with a lid. Simmer until the cauliflower is cooked.
3. Let it cool slightly. Blend with an immersion blender until smooth.
4. Meanwhile, place a saucepan over medium heat. Add oil. When the oil is heated, add onions. Sauté until the onions are translucent.
5. Add mushrooms and cook until the mushrooms are tender.
6. Add the cauliflower puree and bring to the boil. Cover and cook until the soup thickens to the consistency you desire.
7. Serve immediately.

56) Halibut Soup

Serves: 6

Ingredients:

- 2 large onions, chopped
- 2 pounds halibut, chopped into 1 inch chunks
- 2 pounds carrots, peeled, sliced
- 3-4 tablespoons fresh ginger or to taste, peeled, minced
- 2 cups water
- 4 cup chicken broth
- Salt to taste
- Pepper to taste
- 2 tablespoons coconut oil

Method:

1. Place a skillet over medium heat. Add oil. When the oil is melted, add onions and sauté until onions are translucent.
2. Add carrots, broth, ginger and water and bring to the boil.
3. Lower heat and cover with a lid. Simmer for 10-15 minutes or until the vegetables are tender.
4. Remove from heat and blend with an immersion blender until smooth.
5. Place the pot back on heat. Add halibut and simmer without covering until it is tender.
6. Add salt and pepper to taste. Stir well.
7. Ladle into soup bowls and serve.

57) Creamy Cauliflower and Ham Soup

Serves: 5

Ingredients:
- 3 cups cauliflower florets, fresh or frozen (about 12 ounces)
- 1 cup water
- ½ teaspoon onion powder
- ¼ teaspoon garlic powder
- 3 cups ham stock or chicken broth
- 1 ½ cups ham, chopped
- 2 teaspoons fresh thyme leaves, chopped
- 1 tablespoon apple cider vinegar
- 1 tablespoon butter or ghee or bacon fat
- Pepper to taste
- Salt to taste

Method:
1. Place a soup pot over medium heat. Bring to the bowl. Add cauliflower, onion powder, garlic powder, water and stock and stir. Bring to the boil.
2. Lower heat and cover with a lid. Simmer until the cauliflower is cooked.
3. Let it cool slightly. Blend with an immersion blender until smooth.
4. Add ham and thyme leaves and simmer for 7-8 minutes.
5. Add butter and apple cider vinegar and stir. Turn off the heat.
6. Add salt and pepper and stir.
7. Ladle into soup bowls and serve.

58) Easy Green Chicken Enchilada Soup

Serves: 8

Ingredients:

- 1 cup salsa Verde
- 2 cups sharp cheddar cheese, shredded + extra to garnish
- 4 cups chicken, cooked, shredded
- 8 ounces cream cheese, softened
- 4 cups bone broth or chicken stock
- Fresh cilantro, chopped to garnish

Method:

1. Add all the ingredients except chicken into a blender and blend until smooth.
2. Pour into a saucepan. Place the saucepan over medium heat. Let it heat but not boil.
3. Add chicken and heat thoroughly.
4. Ladle into soup bowls. Garnish with cheese and cilantro and serve.

59) Hearty Chicken Stew

Serves: 8

Ingredients:

- 2 pounds chicken breasts, skinless, boneless
- 2 medium carrots, cubed
- 1 small red bell pepper, cut into squares
- 1 small green bell pepper, cut into squares
- 12 fresh mushrooms, quartered
- 1 large tomato, chopped
- 2 stalks celery, chopped
- ½ cup low carb tomato sauce
- 2 teaspoons white pepper powder
- 2 tablespoons coconut oil or ghee
- 4 teaspoons whole peppercorns
- 2 sticks cinnamon
- Salt to taste
- 2 cloves garlic, sliced
- 4 tablespoons butter, unsalted
- 1 bay leaf, crushed
- 6 cups water

Method:

1. Place a large saucepan or pot over medium heat. Add oil and butter. When the butter melts, add cinnamon, peppercorns and bay leaf. After about 5-10 seconds, add garlic and sauté until fragrant.
2. Add onions and sauté until light brown. Add tomatoes and stir. Cook for 2-3 minutes. Stir a couple of times.
3. Add tomato paste and mix again.
4. Lower heat and add water, chicken and all the vegetables except bell peppers. Mix well.
5. Raise the heat to high and bring to the boil.
6. Lower heat and cover with a lid. Simmer until chicken is tender.
7. Uncover and cook for 8-10 minutes.
8. Add bell peppers and cook for 6-7 minutes.
9. Ladle into bowls and serve hot.

60) Chuck Roast Stew

Serves: 4

Ingredients:

- 1-1 ½ pounds grass fed and finished chuck roast, chopped into 2 inch pieces
- ¼ pound uncured bacon, cut into strips
- 1 clove garlic, peeled, smashed
- 1 large red onion, cut into slices
- ½ small green or Savoy cabbage, sliced
- Freshly ground black pepper to taste
- Celtic sea salt to taste
- ½ cup beef broth
- 1 sprig thyme

Method:

1. Place a pot over medium low heat. Add all the ingredients and stir.
2. Cover with a lid. Cook until the meat is tender.
3. Ladle into bowls and serve.

Part 4: Ketogenic Main Course Recipes

61) Crispy Garlic Bombed Parmesan Oven Wings

Serves: 2

Ingredients:

- 10 frozen wings and drums
- 2 tablespoons garlic infused olive oil
- 1 teaspoon garlic powder
- ½ teaspoon garlic salt
- ½ cup parmesan, grated

Method:

1. Let the oven preheat to 450° F.
2. Place the wings on a baking rack. Sprinkle garlic salt. Place the rack in the oven. Place a baking pan below it.
3. Bake for about 30 minutes or until done.
4. Brush garlic oil over it.
5. Broil for 5 minutes until crisp and brown. Remove from the oven and place in a bowl.
6. Pour remaining garlic oil over it and toss well.
7. Sprinkle garlic powder and parmesan and toss well.
8. Serve immediately.

62) Grilled Chicken with Spinach and Melted Mozzarella

Serves: 4

Ingredients:

- 2 large chicken breasts, halved lengthwise to make 4 pieces in all
- 8 ounces frozen spinach, drained
- 1/3 cup roasted red bell pepper, sliced into strips
- 2 cloves garlic, crushed
- 2 ounces part skim mozzarella cheese, shredded
- Salt to taste
- Pepper powder to taste
- 1 teaspoon olive oil
- Cooking spray

Method:

1. Sprinkle salt and pepper over the chicken.
2. Spray a grill or grill pan with cooking spray. Place the chicken and cook for about 3 minutes. Flip sides and cook the other side too. The chicken should not be pink any more.
3. Place a skillet over medium heat. Add oil. When the oil is heated, add garlic and sauté for a few seconds until the garlic is fragrant.
4. Add spinach, salt and pepper and heat thoroughly.
5. Place the grilled chicken on a baking sheet. Divide and place the spinach on top of the chicken.
6. Sprinkle bell pepper and cheese.
7. Let the oven preheat to 400° F.
8. Bake for about 30 minutes and serve.

63) Fettuccine Chicken Alfredo

Serves: 4

Ingredients:

For Alfredo sauce:

- 4 cloves garlic, minced
- 1 cup heavy cream
- 1 teaspoon dried basil
- 4 tablespoons butter
- ½ cup parmesan cheese, grated

For chicken and noodles:

- 2 tablespoons olive oil
- 2 bags Miracle noodle fettuccine noodles
- 4 chicken thighs, skinless, boneless
- Salt to taste
- Pepper to taste

Method:

1. To make Alfredo sauce: Place a pan over low heat. Add butter. When butter melts, add garlic and sauté for a couple of minutes until very light brown.
2. Add parmesan cheese, a little at a time. Add salt, pepper and basil. Stir. When it thickens slightly, add cream and simmer for a couple of minutes. Turn off the heat.
3. Place the chicken thighs on your work area. Pound with a meat mallet until it is about ½ inch thick.
4. Place a pan over medium heat. Add oil. When the oil is heated, add chicken and cook on both the sides for around 7 minutes each.
5. Remove from heat. When cool enough to handle, shred the chicken with a pair of forks. Set aside.
6. Place a large pot of water over medium high heat. Bring to the boil. Drain the water in the noodles from the bag. Rinse in cold water and drain.
7. Add noodles to the boiling water. Boil for 2-3 minutes and drain.
8. Place a large pan or wok over medium heat. When the pan is heated, add the noodles. Spread the noodles all over the pan and cook for a few minutes until dry.
9. Add chicken and Alfredo sauce and toss well. Heat thoroughly and serve.

64) Red Pepper Pesto Chicken in Cucumber Rolls

Serves: 2

Ingredients:

- 1 cup chicken, cooked, shredded
- 2 tablespoons parmesan cheese, shredded (optional)
- 2 cucumbers, halved
- 4 tablespoons low carb pesto of your choice
- 1 small red pepper, chopped
- Pepper to taste
- Salt to taste

Method:

1. Remove the seeds of the cucumber and make like a boat.
2. Mix together all the ingredients except cucumber in a bowl.
3. Stuff the cucumbers with the filling.
4. Serve.

65) Shepherd's Pie

Serves: 3

Ingredients:

- ½ pound ground turkey or lamb or beef
- 2 tablespoons oil
- 1 small onion, chopped
- 1 stalk celery, chopped
- 12 ounces cauliflower rice, cooked
- 2 cloves garlic, minced
- ½ cup tomatoes, chopped
- 2 tablespoons parmesan cheese, grated
- ¼ cup cheese, shredded
- ½ teaspoon dried thyme
- ½ cup heavy cream

Method:

1. Place a skillet over medium heat. Add meat, garlic, onion and celery and sauté until meat is brown.
2. Remove from heat and add tomatoes. Mix well. Spoon the mixture into a casserole dish. Spread it all over the dish.
3. Add cauliflower rice, cream, cheese, parmesan cheese and thyme into a food processor and blend until smooth. Pour over the meat layer in the casserole.
4. Bake in a preheated oven at 350° F for 25-30 minutes.
5. Cool and serve.

66) Eggplant Parmesan Boats

Serves: 6

Ingredients:

- 3 medium eggplants (6 inches each), halved lengthwise
- ¾ pound Italian sausages, discard the casing
- 3 cloves garlic, chopped
- 1 tablespoon olive oil
- 1 medium onion, chopped
- 1/3 cup parmesan cheese, grated
- 1 ½ cups mozzarella cheese, grated
- Salt to taste
- Pepper powder to taste
- 3 cups keto friendly marinara sauce
- ¼ cup basil leaves, chopped

Method:

1. Let the oven preheat to 400° F.
2. Leave around half inch from the edges and scoop the egg plants. Set the scooped part aside.
3. Bake for about 10 - 15 minutes and set aside.
4. Meanwhile, place a skillet over medium heat. Add sausages and onions and cook until the sausages are cooked. Break it simultaneously as it cooks.
5. Add garlic and sauté for a minute.
6. Add the scooped eggplant and stir. Cover and cook until the eggplant is tender.
7. Add about 1 ½ cups marinara sauce, salt and pepper and cook for 3-4 minutes.
8. Turn off the heat.
9. Take a large baking dish. Spread the remaining marinara sauce on the bottom of the dish. Place the baked eggplant cases (with its cut side up).
10. Spoon the eggplant - marinara mixture into the eggplant coverings. Sprinkle sauce.
11. Bake until the cheese melts and light brown in color.
12. Garnish with basil and serve.

67) Cheese Stuffed Bacon Wrapped Hot Dogs

Serves:

Ingredients:

- 20 slices bacon
- 10 hot dogs
- 3 ounces cheddar cheese, chopped into small rectangles
- 1 teaspoon onion powder
- 1 teaspoon garlic powder
- Salt to taste
- Pepper to taste

Method:

1. Slit the hotdogs in the middle leaving the sides intact.
2. Let the oven preheat to 400° F.
3. Gently insert the cheese rectangles inside the slits.
4. Wrap each hot dog tightly with 2 slices of bacon. First place a slice of bacon at one end, insert a toothpick and start wrapping. Place the next slice overlapping the end of the first one. Insert tooth pick on the other end of the hot dog.
5. Repeat the above 2 steps with the remaining hot dogs.
6. Sprinkle salt, pepper, onion, and garlic powder.
7. Place on the rack of the oven.
8. Bake for about 40 minutes or until golden brown.
9. Serve with a keto friendly dip.

68) Low Carb Lasagna Meatballs

Serves: 4
Ingredients:
For the meatballs:

- ½ pound ground chuck
- ½ pound sweet or hot Italian sausage
- 3 tablespoons almond flour
- 1 ½ teaspoons dried parsley
- ¼ teaspoon red pepper flakes
- ¼ teaspoon onion powder or to taste
- ¼ teaspoon garlic powder
- ¼ teaspoon dried oregano
- 1 egg
- ½ teaspoon kosher salt or to taste
- 2 tablespoons parmesan cheese, grated

For the casserole:

- ¾ cup whole milk mozzarella cheese, shredded
- 1 cup keto friendly marinara sauce
- ½ cup whole milk ricotta cheese

Method:

1. Let the oven preheat to 375° F.
2. To make meatballs: Add all the ingredients of the meatballs into a bowl and mix well.
3. Divide the mixture into 16 equal portions. Shape each portion into a ball and place on a baking sheet that is lined with parchment paper.
4. Bake for 15 minutes.
5. To make casserole: Transfer the baked meatballs into a casserole dish.
6. Pour marinara sauce over the balls. Take teaspoons of ricotta cheese and drop it at different spots over the marinara sauce layer.
7. Sprinkle mozzarella cheese all over.
8. Bake for 20-30 minutes. When done, remove from the oven and cool for a few minutes.
9. Serve 4 balls per serving.

69) Parmesan Encrusted Pork Chops

Serves: 6

Ingredients:

- 6 pork chops
- 1 large egg
- 1 cup parmesan cheese, shredded
- 6 tablespoons almond flour
- Salt to taste
- Pepper to taste
- Chili flakes to taste

Method:

1. Mix together in a bowl, parmesan cheese, salt, red chili flakes and pepper.
2. First dip pork chops in egg. Shake to drop off excess egg. Next dredge in the parmesan mixture. Place on a plate.
3. Place a sauté pan over medium heat. Add pork chops and cook on both the sides for a minute each. Cook in batches if required.
4. Remove from the pan and place in a preheated oven. Bake at 400° F for about 10 minutes or until done.

70) Portobello Pizza

Serves: 8

Ingredients:

- 8 large Portobello mushroom caps, cleaned
- 8 ounces fresh mozzarella cheese, cubed
- ¾ cup olive oil
- Pepper to taste
- Salt to taste
- 2 large vine tomatoes, thinly sliced or more if required
- ½ cup fresh basil, chopped
- 40 pepperoni slices

Method:

1. Scrape the inside of the mushroom caps including a little of the flesh to get mushroom shells.
2. Brush generously oil over the mushrooms. Gently rub it into the mushrooms. Sprinkle salt and pepper.
3. Place in a preheated oven and broil for 4-5 minutes. Flip sides and broil the other side too.
4. Remove the mushrooms from the oven and let it cool for a few minutes.
5. To assemble: Place tomato slices over the mushrooms. Sprinkle basil over it.
6. Lay pepperoni slices over the tomatoes alternately (divide the pepperoni and tomato slices among the mushrooms). Sprinkle basil and finally place cheese cubes over it.
7. Place in a preheated oven and broil until the cheese melts and light brown in color.
8. Remove from the oven. Cool for 3-4 minutes and serve.

71) Tasty Beef and Liver Burger

Serves: 8

Ingredients:

- ½ pound chicken livers
- 2 ½ pounds ground beef
- Pepper to taste
- 2 teaspoons sea salt or to taste
- 3 teaspoons ground coriander
- 1 teaspoon red onion, peeled, quartered
- 2 teaspoons poultry seasoning

Method:

1. Add liver and onion into the food processor bowl and pulse until a paste is formed.
2. Add rest of the ingredients and pulse until well combined.
3. Divide the mixture into 8 equal portions.
4. Moisten your hands with water and shape each into patties.
5. Cook on a preheated grill or on a grill pan until done.
6. Serve over lettuce leaves or over keto buns – refer recipe Grilled cheese sandwiches for the buns.

72) Beef Fried Rice

Serves: 3

Ingredients:

- 6 ounces round steak beef
- 2 scallions, sliced into ½ centimeter pieces
- 2 cups cauliflower, grated to rice like texture
- 1 small green bell pepper, chopped
- 2 cloves garlic, sliced
- 1 egg, beaten
- 2 teaspoons olive oil
- 2 tablespoons light soy sauce
- Salt to taste
- Pepper powder to taste

Method:

1. Place a nonstick skillet over medium heat. Add oil. When oil is heated, add garlic and sauté for a few seconds until fragrant.
2. Add scallions and bell pepper and sauté for a minute.
3. Add beef and cook until brown. Turn off the heat.
4. Meanwhile, place another pan over medium heat. Add cauliflower rice to it, cover and cook for 4-5 minutes.
5. Add soy sauce and stir fry for a few seconds. Transfer into the pan of beef. Place the pan back over heat.
6. Add egg and stir. Cook until the eggs are done.
7. Serve hot.

73) Lamb curry

Serves: 2

Ingredients:

- 1 pound lamb, chopped into chunks
- 1 clove garlic, minced
- 1 small tomato, chopped
- 2 tablespoons onion, chopped
- ½ inch piece fresh ginger, minced
- 1 large clove garlic, minced
- 1 cup coconut milk
- 1 teaspoon curry powder
- ¼ teaspoon turmeric powder
- ¼ teaspoon red chili flakes
- ¼ teaspoon ground cumin
- ¼ teaspoon ground ginger
- 1 tablespoon coconut oil
- Fresh cilantro to serve, chopped

Method:

1. Place a saucepan over medium heat. Add oil. When the oil melts, add onion and sauté until onions are translucent.
2. Add garlic and sauté until fragrant. Add tomatoes and all the spices. Sauté for a few minutes until the tomatoes are soft.
3. Increase the heat to high. Add lamb and sauté for a couple of minutes. Add coconut milk and stir.
4. When it begins to boil, lower the heat and cover with a lid. Simmer until the lamb is cooked. Add salt and pepper. Taste and adjust the seasonings if necessary.
5. Serve over cauliflower rice, garnished with cilantro.

74) Double Dipped Coconut Fish Nuggets

Serves: 8

Ingredients:

- 2 pounds fish like cod or snapper or tilapia, rinsed, cut into nuggets
- 1 cup shredded coconut
- 4 eggs, beaten
- Sea salt to taste
- ½ teaspoon pepper powder or to taste
- 1 teaspoon garlic powder
- ¼ - ½ cup coconut oil

Method:

1. Add shredded coconut, salt, garlic powder and pepper powder to a bowl.
2. Dip the nuggets in the egg and then dredge in the coconut mixture and set aside on a plate.
3. Place a skillet over medium heat. Add ¼ cup.
4. Add a few of the nuggets and cook until brown.
5. Repeat step 3 and 4 with the remaining nuggets. Add more oil if required.
6. Serve with any keto friendly dip of your choice.

75) Spicy Tuna Bowl

Serves: 8

Ingredients:

- 2 pounds fresh ahi tuna, chopped into small chunks
- 1 cup edamame, shelled
- 2 bunches scallion, finely chopped
- 4 avocadoes, peeled, pitted, cubed
- 2 bags miracle noodle rice
- 2 tablespoons sesame oil
- 4 tablespoons soy sauce
- 2 jalapeños (optional), finely chopped
- 2 tablespoons black sesame seeds
- 2 tablespoons white sesame seeds
- Salt to taste
- Pepper to taste

For sauce:

- 6 tablespoons mayonnaise
- Juice of a lime
- 2 teaspoons sriracha sauce

Method:

1. Add soy sauce and sesame oil in a bowl and whisk well. Add tuna and toss well. Refrigerate for an hour.
2. Rinse the miracle noodle rice. Place a sauce pan with water over medium heat. Bring to the boil. Add rice and boil for 2 minutes. Drain and transfer rice into a pan.
3. Place the pan over medium heat. Cook until dry.
4. Add all the ingredients including the marinated tuna except sesame seeds into a bowl and toss well. Add sauce and fold gently.
5. Divide into individual serving bowls. Sprinkle sesame seeds over it and serve.

76) Creamy Fish Casserole

Serves: 8

Ingredients:

- 4 tablespoons olive oil
- 12 scallions, finely chopped
- 2 pounds broccoli, cut into small florets, chop the tender stems too
- 3 pounds white fish, chopped into chunks
- 4 tablespoons small capers
- 2 tablespoons dried parsley
- 2 ½ cups heavy whipping cream
- 2 teaspoons salt
- 2 tablespoons Dijon mustard
- ½ teaspoon black pepper
- 7 ounces butter + extra to grease, cubed
- 2 ½ cups heavy whipping cream
- 1 pound leafy greens to serve

Method:

1. Place a skillet over medium high heat. Add oil. When the oil is heated, add broccoli and sauté until it is golden brown in color. Add scallions, capers, salt and pepper. Sauté for a couple of minutes.
2. Transfer half of it into a large greased baking dish. Spread it all over the dish. Place a layer of fish over it. Next layer with the remaining broccoli mixture.
3. Mix together in a bowl, parsley, mustard and cream. Pour over vegetable layer in the baking dish.
4. Place butter cubes all over the dish at different spots.
5. Let the oven preheat to 400°F.
6. Bake for about 20-30 minutes.
7. Serve hot. Serving with a salad made of leafy greens.

77) Creamy Shrimp and Bacon Skillet

Serves: 8

Ingredients:

- 8 slices bacon, chopped into 1 inch pieces
- 8 ounces shelled shrimp, raw
- 8 ounces smoked salmon, cut into strips
- 2 cups mushrooms, sliced
- 1 cup coconut cream or heavy whipping cream
- Freshly ground pepper to taste
- Salt to taste

Method:

1. Place a cast iron skillet over medium heat. Add bacon and cook until tender and not crisp.
2. Add mushrooms and sauté for 4-5 minutes. Stir a couple of times while it is cooking.
3. Increase the heat to high. Add shrimp and cook for a couple of minutes.
4. Add cream, pepper and salt. Lower heat and cook until heated.
5. Serve over miracle noodles or zucchini noodles.

78) Grilled Cheese Sandwich

Serves: 2

Ingredients:

For the keto buns:

- 4 large eggs
- 3 tablespoons psyllium husk powder
- 4 tablespoon butter, softened
- 4 tablespoons almond flour
- 1 teaspoon baking powder

For the sandwich:

- 2 tablespoons butter, for frying
- 4 ounces cheddar cheese

Method:

1. To make keto buns: Add all the ingredients of the bun in a bowl and mix until it becomes thick.
2. Pour half the mixture into a microwave safe square bowl. Make the top of the mixture smooth with a spatula.
3. Microwave on high for 90 seconds or until it is done. Remove from the microwave and remove the bun from the bowl. Cut into 2 halves.
4. Repeat the above 2 steps with the remaining batter.
5. Place a pan over medium heat. Add about a tablespoon of butter.
6. Divide and fill the cheese in 2 halves of the bun. Cover with the other half. Place a sandwich on the pan and fry on both the sides until browned as per you desire.
7. Serve hot.

79) Thai Red Coconut Curry with Broccoli

Serves: 4

Ingredients:

- 2 cups broccoli florets
- 1 medium onion, chopped
- 2 cups fresh spinach
- 2 tablespoons red curry paste
- 2 teaspoons garlic, minced
- 2 teaspoons ginger, minced
- 8 tablespoons coconut oil
- 1 cup thick coconut milk or coconut cream
- 4 teaspoons soy sauce
- 4 teaspoons fish sauce (optional)
- Salt to taste

Method:

1. Place a skillet over medium high heat. Add 3 tablespoons coconut oil. When the oil melts, add onions and sauté until translucent. Add garlic and sauté until light brown.
2. Lower the heat to medium low. Add broccoli and mix well. Cook until broccoli is crisp as well as tender. Push the vegetables to one side of the skillet.
3. Add curry paste and sauté for a few seconds until fragrant.
4. Add spinach and mix the vegetables along with the curry paste. Cook until spinach wilts. Add remaining coconut oil and coconut cream or milk and stir.
5. Add rest of the ingredients and simmer until slightly thick.
6. Serve over cauliflower rice.

80) Spinach Pie

Serves: 8

Ingredients:

- ¼ cup butter
- 2 packages (16 ounces each) frozen chopped spinach, thawed, drained, squeezed of excess moisture
- ¼ cup chopped onions
- 3 cups heavy cream
- 6 eggs
- 1 teaspoon salt
- 1 teaspoon ground nutmeg
- 1 teaspoon black pepper powder
- 1 cup Swiss cheese, shredded

Method:

1. Place a large saucepan over medium heat. Add half the butter. When butter melts, add onions and sauté until the onions are translucent.
2. Add spinach. Cook until the mixture is almost dry. Transfer into a greased pie pan. Sprinkle cheese. Drop about ½ teaspoonful of butter at different spots on the pie.
3. Let the oven preheat to 400°F.
4. Bake for about 20-30 minutes until the top is golden brown.
5. Remove from the oven and cool for 5 minutes.
6. Serve.

Part 5: Ketogenic Dessert Recipes

81) Chocolate Peanut Butter Truffles

Serves: 6

Ingredients:

- 2 tablespoons butter, melted
- 1/2 cup peanut butter
- 3 ounces sugar free chocolate chips
- 3/4 cup powdered xylitol

Method:

1. Add peanut butter, butter and xylitol to a bowl and mix well. If you find the mixture too watery, refrigerate for 30 minutes.
2. Divide the mixture into 6 parts and shape each part into balls. Place on a lined baking sheet.
3. Chill for about 45 minutes.
4. Meanwhile, place chocolate chips to a microwave safe bowl and microwave until melted.
5. Now dip the balls into the melted chocolate. Remove with a slotted spoon and place it back on the lined baking sheet.
6. Chill until the chocolate coating is hardened and serve.

82) Raspberry Panna Cotta

Serves: 8

Ingredients:

- 2 cups almond milk, unsweetened
- 2 cups heavy cream
- 2 sachets unflavored gelatin
- 1/2 cup xylitol or stevia sweetener
- 1 cup sugar free raspberry jam
- 2 tablespoons fresh lemon juice
- 2 teaspoons vanilla extract
- Raspberries to garnish

Method:

1. Place a saucepan over low heat. Add heavy cream and almond milk and stir.
2. Add xylitol and gelatin and heat until the mixture is warm. Do not boil. Whisk until the sweetener is dissolved.
3. Remove from heat. Add vanilla and lemon juice and stir. Pour into 8 greased ramekins.
4. Cover with cling film and chill for at least 4-5 hours.
5. To serve: Run a knife all around the edges of the panna cotta and invert onto a plate.
6. Slice and serve garnished with raspberries

83) Lemon Meringue Mini Tarts

Serves: 8

Ingredients:
For lemon curd:

- 6 egg yolks
- 14 tablespoons butter, cubed
- Juice of 4 lemons
- Zest of 1 lemon, grated
- A pinch xanthan gum
- 20 drops liquid stevia
- 1/2 cup powdered xylitol

For the crust:

- 2 cups almond flour
- 1 egg
- 4 tablespoons whey protein
- 2 tablespoons butter melted
- 4 tablespoons powdered xylitol
- 1/2 teaspoon salt

For meringue:

- 4 tablespoons powdered xylitol
- 4 egg whites
- 1/4 teaspoon cream of tartar

Method:
1. To make the crust: Mix together all the ingredients of the crust using your hands to form a dough.
2. Take 8 tartlet pans (with removable bottom pans) and divide the dough into it. Press the dough into the pans.
3. Bake in a preheated oven 350°F for about 12-15minutes or until light brown. You can bake in batches.
4. Remove from the oven and cool completely.
5. To make lemon curd: Whisk together yolks and xylitol in a heat proof bowl until it becomes pale yellow and place on a double boiler.

6. Cook until the eggs have become thick. Add lemon zest and lemon juice and whisk again.
7. Remove from heat. Add a pinch of xanthan and whisk.
8. Add butter, a little at a time beat with an electric mixer until creamy beating each time. When all the butter is added, chill in the refrigerator for a while.
9. To make meringue: Add egg whites to a mixing bowl and beat with an electric mixer until it doubles in volume.
10. Add cream of tartar and whip again. Add xylitol, a little at a time beating on medium speed each time simultaneously.
11. Beat on high speed until stiff peaks are formed.
12. To assemble: Divide and spread the lemon curd on top of the crusts. Place a spoonful of meringue.
13. Bake in a preheated oven 350°F for about 12-15minutes golden brown.

84) Blueberry Mousse

Serves: 12

Ingredients:

- 3 cups blueberries
- 3 cups firm tofu, drained, crumbled
- 1 cup heavy cream
- 5 tablespoons xylitol or stevia sweetener
- Dark dairy-free chocolate, shaved to serve

Method:

1. Add blueberries to the blender and blend.
2. Add tofu and blend until smooth. Add sweetener and cream and blend until well combined.
3. Transfer into individual serving bowls. Refrigerate for 3-4 hours before serving.
4. Serve garnished with chocolate shavings and a few blueberries.

85) Strawberry Shortcake

Serves: 20
Ingredients:
For shortcakes:

- 6 ounces cream cheese
- 4 tablespoons xylitol
- 6 large eggs, separated
- 1 teaspoon vanilla extract
- 1/2 teaspoon baking powder

For filling:

- 2 cups whipped cream
- 20 medium strawberries, sliced

Method:
1. Beat egg whites until light and fluffy.
2. Add cream cheese to the yolks along with vanilla extract, xylitol, and baking powder. Beat until smooth and creamy.
3. Add whites and fold lightly into the cream cheese mixture.
4. Grease 2-3 large baking sheets. Line with parchment paper.
5. Drop large spoonfuls on the baking sheet. Leave space between 2 shortcakes.
6. Bake in a preheated oven 300°F for about 25 minutes. You can bake in batches.
7. Spread whipped cream on all the shortcakes. Lay strawberry slices on half the shortcakes. Cover with the remaining shortcakes.

86) Chocolate Cake in a mug

Serves: 2

Ingredients:

- 4 tablespoons cocoa powder
- 4 tablespoons xylitol or sugar substitute of choice or to taste
- A pinch salt
- 2 tablespoons heavy cream
- 1 teaspoon vanilla extract
- 1/2 teaspoon baking powder
- Whipped cream to serve
- Berries of your choice to serve
- Cooking spray

Method:

1. Mix together all the dry ingredients in a bowl.
2. Add cream, vanilla, and egg and mix well.
3. Spray the mugs with cooking spray.
4. Pour into mugs (1/2 fill it).
5. Microwave on high for about 60-80 seconds or until the top of the cake is slightly hard.
6. Cool and invert on to a plate. Serve with whipped cream and berries.

87) Strawberry Basil Ice Cups

Serves: 5
Method:

- 6 tablespoons cream cheese
- 4 tablespoons creamed coconut milk
- 2 tablespoons butter, unsalted, at room temperature
- 2 tablespoons powdered xylitol or stevia
- Liquid stevia drops to taste (optional)
- A handful fresh basil leaves
- 1/2 cup fresh strawberries + extra to garnish
- 1/2 teaspoon vanilla extract
-

Method:

1. Add all the ingredients except strawberries and basil to a blender and blend until smooth.
2. Remove half the blended mixture and set aside.
3. To the other half that is in the blender add strawberries and blend until smooth.
4. Divide the mixture into 5 silicone muffin cups.
5. Clean the blender and add the blended mixture that was set aside. Add basil leaves and blend until smooth.
6. Divide the mixture and spoon into the muffin cups above the strawberry layer.
7. Place thinly sliced strawberry slices on top.
8. Freeze for a few hours until set.

88) Blueberry Ice cream

Serves: 6

Ingredients:

- 3/4 cup crème fraiche
- 3/4 cup blueberries, fresh or frozen
- 1 1/2 cups heavy cream
- 1 tablespoon vanilla protein powder
- 2 yolks

Method:

1. Whip cream in a bowl until slightly fluffy.
2. Whip crème fraiche in another larger bowl until slightly fluffy.
3. Add most of the whipped cream to it. Also add yolk, and most of the blueberries and whip well.
4. Freeze for an hour.
5. Serve in individual dessert bowls. Dot with remaining whipped cream and sprinkle the remaining blueberries.

89) Apple-Apricot Cloud

Serves: 12

Ingredients:

- 32 ounces apple-apricot sauce, unsweetened
- 3 cups heavy cream
- 4 tablespoons xylitol or stevia sweetener

Method:

1. Add cream and xylitol to the mixing bowl and beat with an electric mixer until firm peaks are formed.
2. Add apple-apricot sauce and fold gently.
3. Transfer into 8 dessert bowls.
4. Chill and serve later.

90) Creamy Peanut Butter Dessert

Serves: 4

Ingredients:

- 6 tablespoons peanut butter, unsalted
- Sweetener of your choice
- 1/2 cup whipped cream
- 1 tablespoon cocoa powder

Method:

1. Divide the peanut butter and place in 4 individual bowls (about 1 1/2 tablespoons)
2. Sprinkle sweetener over it.
3. Spread some cream over the peanut butter.
4. Sprinkle cocoa powder over the cream.
5. Divide the remaining cream (if it is remaining) amongst the bowls and serve.

91) Lime Mousse

Serves: 8

Ingredients:

- 2 cups heavy cream
- 4 ounces cream cheese
- 7-8 tablespoons xylitol or stevia sweetener or to taste
- 2 teaspoons coconut extract or vanilla extract
- 1/2 cup fresh lime juice
- Coconut flakes to garnish, unsweetened (optional)

Method:

1. Add cream cheese to the mixing bowl and beat with an electric mixer until smooth and creamy.
2. Add xylitol and beat until well blended. Add lime juice and beat again.
3. Add coconut extract and heavy cream and beat until well blended
4. Transfer into individual 8 dessert bowls.
5. Garnish with coconut flakes.
6. Chill and serve later

92) Rich Chocolate Muffin

Serves: 4

Ingredients

- 3 cups almond flour
- 2 cups heavy cream
- 3 large eggs
- 1 cup melted butter
- 1 cup xylitol
- 2 tsp. vanilla extract
- 2 tsp. baking soda
- ½ tsp. salt
- 1 cup chocolate chips (ensure that the brand you choose has low carbohydrates)

Method

1. Preheat the oven to 300degrees Fahrenheit.
2. Keep the muffin covers in each hole of the muffin pan.
3. Take a small bowl and add the cream and the almond flour. Whisk the two ingredients together.
4. Add the eggs one at a time and keep stirring till the mixture has become smooth.
5. Add the butter, baking soda, sweetener, flavoring and the salt to the bowl. Mix all the ingredients together.
6. Add the chocolate to the bowl and stir the ingredients together till they are distributed evenly.
7. Take the mixture and place it in each of the muffin holes. Bake the cupcakes for thirty minutes. Leave them in the oven till they are golden brown.
8. Let them cool down. Serve them with butter.

93) Chocolate Cherry Cheesecake

Serves: 6

Ingredients

- 16 ounces cream cheese (softened at room temperature)
- 4 ounces heavy cream
- 2 tsp. Stevia Glycerite
- 2 tsp. Splenda (or any other artificial sweetener which is low in carbohydrates)
- 2 tbsp. Dutch processed cocoa powder
- 2 tbsp. Sugar free cherry syrup

Method

- Add all the ingredients in a large mixing bowl.
- Whisk them well until it has a pudding like consistency.
- Spoon the batter into small cups and leave it in the refrigerator to set.

94) Cinnamon Churritos:

Serves: 8

Ingredients:

- 3 cups almond flour
- 1/3 cup coconut flour
- 3/4 teaspoon baking powder
- 6 teaspoons ground cinnamon, divided
- 1/2 teaspoon salt
- 3/4 cup coconut milk
- 3 tablespoons unsalted butter
- 6 tablespoons granular sugar substitute like xylitol, divided
- 3 large eggs
- Oil for deep frying

Method:

1. Place oil for deep-frying in a shallow skillet or a deep fryer. Oil should cover at least 2-3 inches height from the bottom of the skillet. Heat oil to 375-degree F.
2. Meanwhile make the dry mixture as follows: Mix together almond flour, coconut flour, baking powder, half the cinnamon and salt. Keep aside
3. Place a saucepan over medium heat. Pour the coconut milk. Add butter, and 3 tablespoons xylitol. Bring to a boil.
4. Remove from heat. Add the dry mixture to this and mix well until it is thick and resembles a dough.
5. Let it cool for 10 minutes.
6. Add the eggs and mix again to form a thick paste.
7. Drop tablespoons of this mixture into the hot oil. About 5-6 per batch. Fry until golden brown.
8. Turn the Churritos on all sides so that it is evenly brown.
9. Remove with a slotted spoon and place on paper towels until the next batch is ready.
10. Repeat step 7 - 9 with the remaining batter.
11. Pulse together the xylitol and cinnamon in a blender to make the xylitol granules slightly finer. Transfer on to a plate.
12. Roll the fried Churritos over the xylitol – cinnamon mixture. Coat well.
13. Serve immediately if you like it hot or serve it at room temperature

95) Vanilla Crème Pudding Parfaits

Serves: 8

Ingredients:

- 2 cans (14.5 ounces each) full fat coconut milk, chilled
- 2 teaspoons vanilla extract
- 20 drops liquid stevia
- 1/2 cup walnuts, chopped
- 1 1/2 cups fresh berries of your choice
- Ground cinnamon to garnish

Method:

1. To make vanilla crème: Pour coconut milk to the bowl of your stand mixer. Add stevia and vanilla extract. Whisk until well combined.
2. Add berries and walnuts to a bowl. Toss well.
3. Take 8 parfait glasses. Add about 3 spoonsful of vanilla crème into each of the glasses.
4. Use about 1/2 the berry mixture and layer over the vanilla crème.
5. Next layer with the remaining vanilla crème followed by the remaining half of the berry mixture.
6. Sprinkle ground cinnamon on top and serve.

96) Pumpkin Spice Crème Brule

Serves: 6

Ingredients:

- 4 egg yolks
- 2 cups heavy cream
- 4 tablespoons pumpkin puree
- 2 teaspoons pumpkin pie spice
- 4 tablespoons xylitol + extra for sprinkling

Method:

1. Place a heavy bottomed pan on low heat. Add cream and heat.
2. Once it starts bubbling, remove from heat. Add pumpkin pie spice and stir. Cover and set aside for 5 minutes.
3. Whisk the yolks until light yellow in color.
4. Add about a tablespoon of the cream mixture to the eggs and whisk constantly. Continue this process until all the cream is added.
5. Add pumpkin puree and whisk again. Add xylitol and stir until well combined.
6. Transfer into 6 ramekins. Take a large baking dish. Pour enough hot water to cover 1 inch from the bottom of the dish.
7. Place the ramekins inside the baking dish.
8. Bake in a preheated oven at 250°F for about 45 minutes or until set.
9. Remove from the oven and cool.
10. Sprinkle xylitol.
11. Serve either chilled or at room temperature.

97) Strawberry Cheesecake Fat Bombs

Serves: 5

Ingredients:

- 1 1/2 cups cream cheese, at room temperature,
- 1 cup strawberries, fresh or frozen
- 1/2 cup butter, chopped into small pieces, softened
- 1 tablespoon vanilla extract
- 30 drops liquid stevia or 4 tablespoons xylitol

Method:

1. Add softened butter and cream cheese to a bowl and mix until well combined.
2. Add the strawberries, vanilla and stevia to a blender and blend until smooth. Transfer into the bowl of cream cheese. Whisk well.
3. Transfer the mixture into candy molds or small muffin molds.
4. Chill until set and serve.

98) Lemon Cheesecake Pudding

Serves: 4

Ingredients:

- 12 ounces of softened cream cheese
- 3/4 cup heavy cream
- 6 -7 packets of artificial sweetener
- 1 teaspoon lemon extract

Method:

1. Blend together all the ingredients until smooth and pour into individual dessert bowls.
2. Chill and serve later.

99) Mocha Ice cream

Serves: 6

Ingredients:

- 2 cups coconut milk
- 1 cup heavy cream
- 1/4 cup xylitol
- 30 drops liquid stevia
- 1/4 cup cocoa powder
- 2 tablespoons instant coffee
- 1/2 teaspoon. Xanthan Gum

Method:

1. Mix together all the ingredients except xanthan gum in a mixing bowl. With a stick blender, blend the ingredients.
2. Add the xanthan gum little by little, blending continuously.
3. Freeze the ice cream for 5-6 hours or until set. Remove from the freezer around 30 minutes before serving.
4. Serve sprinkled with a little instant coffee. Alternately, you can freeze in an ice cream maker following the manufacturer's instructions.

100) Mint and Chocolate Chip Ice Bombs

Serves: 6

Ingredients:

- 1/2 cup full fat mascarpone cheese or creamed coconut milk
- 1 ounce 90 % dark chocolate, chopped
- 2 1/2 tablespoons powdered xylitol or stevia
- Liquid stevia drops to taste (optional)
- 1/2 teaspoon peppermint extract or 2 teaspoons fresh mint, minced

Method:

1. Add all the ingredients to a blender and blend until smooth.
2. Add about 2 tablespoons of the mixture into round molds or small silicone muffin molds.
3. Freeze until set